Radio / Phone Consultation

Identify: Unit #	Your Name
Patient Age	Sex

Chief Complaint (onset, duration, etc)	

LOC	Level of Distress

Signs & Symptoms	

Pulse	BP
Respirations	Other
Skin	Pupils
Lung sounds	EKG
Past Medical HX	
Medications	
Allergies	
Physician	
Emergency care	
ETA	En route code
Time	Other

D1767059

2

Airway

Rapid Sequence Intubation

1 **Prepare equipment** (IV, ECG, oximeter, BVM, suction, ETT)

2 **C-Spine Immobilization p.r.n.**

3 **Preoxygenate with 100% O_2**

4 If suspected ↑ICP:
- **Give Lidocaine 1.5 mg/kg IV**

5 **Give Sedative:**
- Midazolam 0.1–0.3 mg/kg IV or
- Thiopental 1–3 mg/kg IV or
- Ketamine 1–2 mg/kg IV or
- Etomidate 0.3 mg/kg IV or
- Diazepam 0.2 mg/kg IV (max 20 mg)

6 If pt < 2 y.o., **give Atropine 0.02 mg/kg IV**
- (blocks reflex bradycardia)

7 **Give Succinylcholine 1–1.5 mg/kg IV**
- *or:* **Rocuronium 0.6–1.2 mg/kg IV**
- *or:* **Vecuronium 0.1 mg/kg IV**

8 **Intubate**
- (apply cricoid pressure p.r.n.)

9 **Inflate Cuff / Verify Tube Placement:**
- Check Chest Expansion
- Check Lung Sounds
- Fogging of tube
- Apply CO2 Detector
- Secure c̄ ETT holder & C-collar

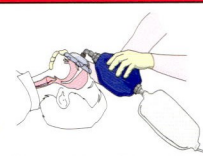

Place pt in sniff position. Hyperventilate with O_2

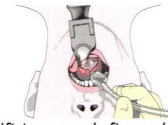

Lift tongue leftward & visualize vocal cords

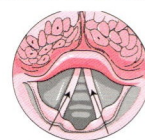

Vocal cords

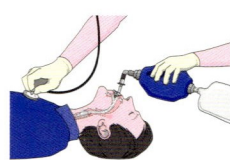

Insert ETT; inflate cuff; check breath sounds

Laryngeal Mask Airway

Contra—Severe oropharyngeal trauma; **poorly tolerated in conscious pts**

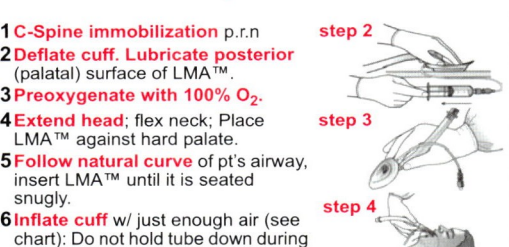

1 **C-Spine immobilization** p.r.n
2 **Deflate cuff. Lubricate posterior** (palatal) surface of LMA™.

step 2

3 **Preoxygenate with 100% O_2.**
4 **Extend head**; flex neck; Place LMA™ against hard palate.

step 3

5 **Follow natural curve** of pt's airway, insert LMA™ until it is seated snugly.
6 **Inflate cuff** w/ just enough air (see chart): Do not hold tube down during inflation; allow LMA™ to "seat itself".

step 4

7 **Verify proper placement:**
   ✓ Check Cx expansion & lung Sounds
   ✓ Secure with tape or tube holder

step 5

   ✓ Apply CO_2 detector; oximeter
   ✓ Reassess airway periodically

Illustrations © 2003 LMA North America, Inc.

step 6

Patient Size	LMA™ Size	Max Cuff Vol.
Neonate/Infant: up to 5 kg	1	up to 4 ml
Infant: 5–10 kg	1 ½	up to 7 ml
Infant/Child: 10–20 kg	2	up to 10 ml
Child: 20–30 kg	2 ½	up to 14 ml
Child: 30–50 kg	3	up to 20 ml
Normal Adult: 50–70 kg	4	up to 30 ml
Large Adult: 70–100 kg	5	up to 40 ml
Large Adult: > 100 kg	6	up to 50 ml

Combitube®

Contra— Gag reflex, esophageal disease, caustic ingestion, under 16 y.o. or < 5' tall (use Combitube SA® for small adult).

1 Immobilize C-spine if spinal trauma; Hyperventilate with 100% O₂—apply cricoid pressure p.r.n.

2 Prepare equipment
Combitube, suction, oximeter.

3 Place head in neutral position.
Open pt's mouth with jaw lift; Insert device to markings on tube. Teeth should be between black markings (A).

4 Inflate pharyngeal cuff (#1) with 100cc air (B).

5 Inflate distal cuff (#2) with 15cc air (C).

6 Ventilate through longer, blue tube (#1).
Auscultate lungs & stomach; If lung sounds are present:

7 Continue ventilation through blue tube.

8 If gastric sounds are heard (and no lung sounds), **ventilate through short, clear tube** (#2). Verify lung sounds.

9 If present, continue ventilation through short, clear tube #2

10 Secure tube with tape. Reassess airway periodically.

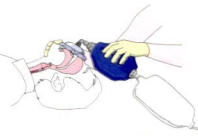

Hyperventilate c̄ O₂

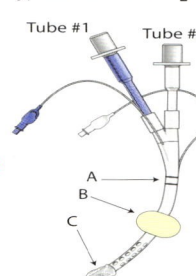

Tube #1   Tube #2

A
B
C

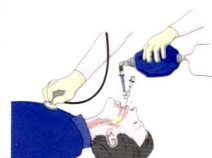

Check breath sounds

King LT™ Airway

Contra—Patients < 4 feet. Does not protect against aspiration.

1. **C-Spine Immobilization** p.r.n. Preoxygenate with 100% O_2.
2. **Deflate cuff. Open mouth, apply chin lift, insert tip** into side of mouth.
3. **Advance tip** behind tongue while rotating tube to midline.
4. **Advance tube** until base of connector is aligned with teeth or gums.
5. **Inflate cuff** with air: (use minimum volume necessary).

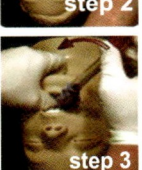

step 2

Pt Size	LT Size	Cuff Vol
4-5 feet	Size 3	45-60 ml
5-6 feet	Size 4	60-80 ml
> 6 feet	Size 5	70-90 ml

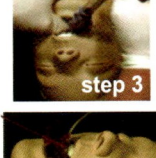

step 3

6. **Attach Bag-Valve device**. While ventilating, gently withdraw tube until ventilation becomes easy.
7. **Adjust cuff inflation** if necessary to obtain a good seal.
8. **Verify Proper Placement**:
   - Check Cx Expansion & Lung Sounds
   - Apply CO_2 Detector; oximeter
   - Secure with tape or tube holder
   - Reassess airway periodically

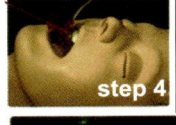

step 4

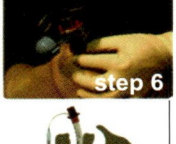

step 6

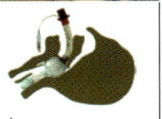

(illustrations © 2005 King Systems, Inc.)

Trauma Triage Criteria
(For Patient Entry into the Trauma System)

PHYSIOLOGICAL
- Systolic BP **less than 90 mm/Hg**
- Respiratory Distress—Rate < 10 or > 29
- Altered mental status, or Glasgow Coma Score ≤ 13

ANATOMICAL
- Flail chest
- Two or more proximal long bone fractures (humerus, femur)
- Penetrating injury to the head, neck, torso or groin that is associated with significant energy transfer (bullet, knife, impalement, etc.)
- Partial or full thickness burns to the face or airway
- Amputation proximal to the wrist or ankle
- Paralysis of any limb associated with trauma injury

MECHANISM
- Extrication taking > 20 minutes using heavy tools
- Death of any occupant in the patient's vehicle
- Ejection of patient from an enclosed vehicle
- Falls greater than 15 feet

COMORBID FACTORS
(any combination of high-energy transfer in comorbid factor should increase the index of suspicion for severe trauma injury)
- **Age < 12 or > 60**
- Pregnancy
- Significant preexisting medical problems
- Extremes of environment: Hot or Cold
- Presence of Intoxicant

INDEX OF SUSPICION— The reason for system entry must be fully documented. You may enter any patient into the Trauma System suspected of having experienced significant trauma regardless of physical findings. Any combination of comorbid factors and high energy transfer is dangerous.

Rapid Triage (Multiple Patient Scenes)

Priority	Color	Condition	Notes
1	Red	Immediate	Life threatening
2	Yellow	Urgent	Can delay up to 1 h
3	Green	Delayed	Up to 3 hours
4	Black	Deceased	No care needed

Priority 1—Immediate Transport

Unconscious, disoriented, very confused, rapid respirations, weak irregular pulse, severe uncontrolled bleeding, other signs of shock (cold, clammy skin, low blood pressure, etc.)

Priority 2—Urgent Can Delay Transport up to 1 hr

Conscious, oriented, with any significant fracture or other significant injury, but without signs of shock.

Priority 3—Delayed Transport up to 3 hrs

Walking wounded, CAO x3, minor injuries.

Priority 4—Deceased, No Care Needed

No pulse, no respirations (open airway first), obvious mortal wounds (e.g. decapitation).

NOTES: Assessment of patients should be < 1 minute each.
(Have someone else control bleeding during your survey.)
- All unconscious patients are RED—Immediate
- "Walking wounded" are usually GREEN—Priority 3
- All pulseless patients are BLACK—Priority 4

Mentation / LOC Assessment

▼A—Alert: able to answer questions

▼V—Verbal: responds to verbal stimuli

▼P—Pain: responds only to pain stimuli. Protect airway

▼U—Unconscious: protect airway, consider intubation

8

Multiple Patients

1 **Strategically park vehicle and stay in one place.**

2 **Establish Command,** and identify yourself as Command to dispatch (use a calm, clear voice).

3 **Size up the scene** and advise dispatch of:
   - Exact location and type of incident
   - Any hazardous conditions
   - The location of the command post
   - The best routes of access to the scene
   - Estimated number and severity of patients

4 **Designate an EMT to perform rapid triage** (*see* **Rapid Triage** on page 8), tag and number multiple patients ("**Immediate**", "**Urgent**", "**Delayed**")

5 **Order resources** (Fire, Police, Ambulances, HazMat, Extrication, Air Units, Tow vehicles, Buses, etc.).

6 **Set up staging areas** (clearly state the location of staging/assembly areas, and think of access and egress).

7 **Coordinate access** of incoming units to the scene.

8 **Assign patients to incoming medical units.**
9 **Maintain communications with On Line Medical Control (OLMC).**

10 **Keep patient log** indicating patient number, severity, treating and transporting units, medical interventions, and destination hospitals.

Mass Casualty Incident

Use Multiple Patient guidelines + the following ICS groups

Medical Branch Director

- Responsible for overall medical direction / coordination
- Orders additional medical resources
- Serves as a resource for group supervisors

Triage Group Supervisor

- Estimates number and severity of patients
- Establishes tagging and extrication teams
- Establishes triage areas, if necessary
- Maintains rapid and orderly flow of patients to treatment areas

Treatment Area Supervisor

- Secures treatment areas, identifies equipment needs
  - Clearly marks Treatment Areas for **"Immediate"**, **"Urgent"**, **"Delayed"**
- Establishes treatment teams when resources allow.
- Identifies order of patient transport

Transportation Group Supervisor

- Establishes Patient Loading Zone (near Treatment Area)
- Assigns patients to ambulances, supervises actual loading
- Relays Unit number, severity and number of patients to Communications Group Supervisor

Communications Group Supervisor

- Communicates with On-Line Medical Control (OLMC) to identify receiving hospitals
- Maintains patient log
- Receives information from Transportation Group
- Coordinates patient destinations to avoid overloading the closest hospitals

Burn Chart

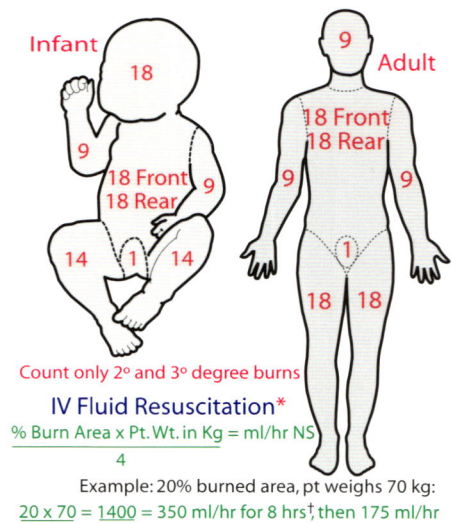

Infant

Adult

18

9

9

18 Front
18 Rear

9

14

1

14

9

18 Front
18 Rear

9

9

1

18

18

Count only 2° and 3° degree burns

IV Fluid Resuscitation*

$$\frac{\% \text{ Burn Area x Pt. Wt. in Kg}}{4} = \text{ml/hr NS}$$

Example: 20% burned area, pt weighs 70 kg:

$$\frac{20 \times 70}{4} = \frac{1400}{4} = 350 \text{ ml/hr for 8 hrs†, then 175 ml/hr}$$
over the next 16 hrs.

† calculated from the time of injury

* Patients in shock need more aggressive IV fluid replacement
and should be treated according to your shock protocol.

**Major burns should be treated in a burn center,
including: ≥ 25% body surface; hands, feet, face or
perineum; electrical burns; inhalation burns; other
injuries; or severe preexisting medical problems.**

Trauma—Abdominal

HX—Mechanism of injury, associated trauma, penetrating vs blunt injury? Suspect internal hemorrhage. **Guarding, distension, rigidity, hypotension, pallor, bruising?**
RUQ: liver, gall bladder, duodenum, head of pancreas, right kidney (posteriorly), ascending colon, transverse colon.
LUQ: stomach, tail of pancreas, liver, left kidney (posteriorly), spleen, transverse colon, descending colon.
LLQ: small intestine, descending colon, left ovary, fallopian tube.
RLQ: appendix, cecum, right ovary, fallopian tube, small intestine.
Midline: great vessels (aorta, vena cava), bladder, uterus.
Back: kidneys, spleen on L side.
❖**Vitals, O₂, *IV*, treat for shock, transport.**

Trauma—Chest

Suspect cardiac, pulmonary, or great vessel trauma.

HX—MOI: estimate forces involved. Lung disease?
Respiratory distress? Pain? **Use of accessory muscles?** Level of consciousness, color? GCS? Is patient anxious? **Tracheal shift?** Symmetrical cx expansion? JVD? Lung sounds? **Hemoptysis? Sub-Q emphysema &/or crepitus?**
Life threatening chest injuries:
• Flail segment
• Open chest wounds
• Tension pneumothorax
❖**Secure airway, high flow O₂, intubate if necessary and assist ventilations.**
❖**Open chest wound:** cover with occlusive dressing. Look for exit wounds.
❖**Tension pneumothorax:** Evaluate and decompress.
❖**Impaled objects**: stabilize in place. Do not delay transport if patient is unstable. *Consider IV fluids for shock (2 large bore IVs), Monitor EKG, Vitals. Full spinal immobilization.*
Caution—Consider other causes for respiratory distress.

Trauma—General

HX— mechanism of injury, location of trauma, penetrating vs blunt injury? Assess level of consciousness (Alert, Verbal, Pain, Unconscious). **Airway obstruction?** Pulses, BP, capillary refill; severe bleeding? Disability / neuro assessment, Glasgow coma score, Expose and perform exam, Check pupils; **tracheal deviation?** Sub-Q air? Jugular venous distension? **Assess chest:** look for trauma, pneumo, check lung sounds, Evaluate abdomen, pelvis, extremities, back. Abdominal guarding, distension, rigidity, **hypotension,** pallor, bruising? Are there medical causes? (e.g. diabetes, CVA, MI, etc.)
❖**Assess scene safety.** Protect C-Spine; Give O₂, Check respiratory rate, adequacy—ventilate if needed.

Trauma—Head

❖**HX**— MOI, estimate forces involved. Any changes in LOC? Amnesia? Was seat belt, helmet worn? Respiratory rate, pattern, quality; Chest or trunk injuries? Vitals, Pupils, Neuro deficits? Posturing? Reflexes? Blood or CSF from ears, nose? Scalp, skull depression, associated facial trauma?
❖Secure airway while providing C-spine immobilization. Control bleeding with direct pressure. Do not stop bleeding from nose, ears if CSF leak is suspected. Give O₂, *Start large bore IV (TKO unless patient is in shock).* Monitor vitals & neuro status. *EKG,* Pulse oximetry; *Consider intubation and ventilation if GCS ≤ 8*
❖**Caution**— Always suspect C-spine injury in the head injury patient. Assess and document LOC changes. Be alert for airway problems and seizures. Restlessness & or agitation can be due to hypoxia or hypoglycemia. Check chemstrip.

Traumatic Cardiac Arrest

Penetrating trauma? Transport rapidly to trauma center.

HX—Mechanism of injury, associated trauma, penetrating vs. blunt injury? Any vital signs upon arrival? **If blunt trauma (MVA, crush injury) survival = < 1%;** consider pronouncing patient dead in the field, especially if there are other patients who need medical care (contact OLMC).

❖**Rapid extrication and transport immediately. Secure airway, do CPR (shock VF). O₂, IVs, en route. Splint fractures en route.**

Glasgow Coma Scale

INFANT	Eye Opening		CHILD/ADULT
4	Spontaneously	Spontaneously	4
3	To Speech	To Command	3
2	To Pain	To Pain	2
1	No Response	No Response	1
	Best Verbal Response		
5	Coos, babbles	Oriented	5
4	Irritable cries	Confused	4
3	Cries to pain	Inappropriate words	3
2	Moans, grunts	Incomprehensible	2
1	No Response	No Response	1
	Best Motor Response		
6	Spontaneous	Spontaneous	6
5	Localizes pain	Localizes pain	5
4	Withdraws from pain	Withdraws from pain	4
3	Flexion (decorticate)	Flexion (decorticate)	3
2	Extension (decerebrate)	Extension (decerebrate)	2
1	No Response	No Response	1

___**= TOTAL →(GCS ≤ 8? → Intubate!) ←TOTAL=**___

Pediatric Trauma Score

	+2		-1	score
Pt Size	> 20 kg	10 – 20 kg	< 10 kg	
Airway	Normal	Maintainable s̄ invasive procedures	Not maintainable: NEEDS invasive procedures	
CNS	Awake	Obtunded	Comatose	
Systolic BP (or pulse)	> 90 (radial)	50 – 90 (femoral)	< 50 mm Hg (no pulse)	
Open Wounds	None	Minor	Major or Penetrating	
Skeletal	None	Closed Fx	Open / Multiple Fx	

+12 = Minimal or no injury
≤ 8 = Critical injury: transport to pediatric trauma center

Total =

ACLS Algorithms

NOTE: Not all patients require the treatment indicated by these algorithms. They assume that you have assessed the patient, started CPR where indicated, and performed reassessment after each treatment. They also do not exclude other appropriate interventions which may be warranted by the patient's condition. **Treat the patient, not the ECG.**

Treatment Classes—Risks vs. Benefits

Class I: Benefit>>>Risk: **should be performed**
Class IIa: Benefit>>Risk: **a reasonable treatment**
Class IIb: Benefit>Risk: **may be considered**
Class Indeterminate: insufficient evidence—**no recommendations**
Class III: Risk > Benefit: not helpful, may be harmful

Possible Causes of Cardiac Arrest/Arrhythmia

Hypoxia—Ventilation
Hypovolemia—IV Fluids
Hypothermia—Warm patient
Hypokalemia—Restore electrolyte balance
Hypoglycemia—Dextrose
Hypothermia—Warm patient
Toxins—Detoxify & appropriate therapies
Coronary or Pulmonary Thrombosis—Thrombolysis
Trauma—Surgery / Control Hemorrhage
Cardiac Tamponade—Pericardiocentesis
Tension Pneumothorax—Thoracic Decompression
Hyperkalemia—Sodium Bicarbonate 1 mEq/kg IV
Metabolic Acidosis—▼Sodium Bicarbonate 1 mEq/kg IV
Respiratory Acidosis—Ventilation

Special Footnotes

▼**Sodium bicarbonate (1 mEq/kg IV) is Class IIa:**
For metabolic acidosis, hyperkalmia, or TCA overdose
Class IIb: for prolonged cardiac arrest & for some toxidromes;
Sodium bicarbonate is contraindicated (Class III)
in hypercarbic acidosis (arrest with pt not intubated).

Pulseless Arrest—V-Fib / V-Tach

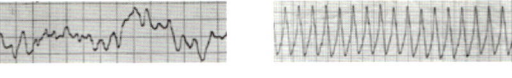

Assess ABCs, Perform CPR (30:2, 100/min)

✔ **Defibrillate @ 120–200 J Biphasic energy**
(or 360J monophasic energy, or AED)

Continue CPR Immediately x 5 Cycles (2 minutes)

Asystole? PEA?
—*See* Asystole / PEA
Algorithm page 19

Pulse Present?
Assess vital signs
Support airway &
breathing
Give meds appropriate
for BP, HR and ECG.

Still VF / VT?

✔ **Defibrillate 120–200J** (or 360J monophasic, or AED)
Continue CPR Immediately x 5 Cycles (~2 minutes)

Intubate (verify ETT placement and secure tube), Start IV/IO
Epinephrine 1 mg IV/IO—repeat q̄ 3–5 minutes, *OR:*
Vasopressin 40 U IV/IO (single dose only)
(▼**Sodium bicarbonate** (1 mEq/kg) if patient is hyperkalemic)

Still VF / VT?

✔ **Defibrillate 120–200J** (or 360J monophasic, or AED)
Continue CPR Immediately x 5 Cycles (~2 minutes)

Amiodarone 300 mg IV/IO, (may repeat once 150 mg in 5 min) *OR:*
Lidocaine 1 – 1.5 mg/kg IV/IO,
(may give 0.5 – 0.75 mg/kg in 5 min. x3 or max 3 mg/kg) *OR:*
Magnesium sulfate 1 – 2 Gm IV/IO,
(for torsades de pointes, hypomagnesemia)

Still VF / VT?

✔ **Defibrillate 120 – 200J** (or 360J monophasic, or AED)
Continue CPR Immediately x 5 Cycles (~2 minutes)

Epinephrine 1 mg IV/IO—repeat q̄ 3–5 minutes
▼**See Special Footnotes, page 16**

Electrical Cardioversion

(for non-arrest tachycardia, with serious signs and symptoms related to the tachycardia)

If ventricular rate is > 150 beats / minute
(Immediate cardioversion is usually not needed for rates <150)

↓

Check O_2 saturation
Prepare suction, IV, Intubation equipment
Premedicate whenever possible
(Consider anesthesia if readily available: **diazepam, midazolam, barbiturates, etomidate, ketamine, methohexital, propofol**)

✔ **Synchronized BIPHASIC cardioversion for:**

VT 75 J → 120 J → 150 J → 200 J
(Treat polymorphic VT [irregular form & rate] like VF: 120 → 200J Biphasic or 360J Monophasic)
Atrial fibrillation: 30 J → 50 J → 75 J → 120 J
PSVT/Atrial flutter: 30J → 50J → 75 J → 120 J
Sample energies: **use energies that are specific to your defibrillator.** If delays in synchronization occur and patient is critical, **administer immediate unsynchronized shocks.**

✔ **Synchronized MONOPHASIC cardioversion for:**

VT 100J → 200J → 300J → 360J
(Treat polymorphic VT [irregular form & rate] like VF: 360J monophasic)
Atrial fibrillation: 100J → 200J →300J → 360J
PSVT/Atrial Flutter: 50J → 100J → 200J → 300J → 360J

Synchronize Markers

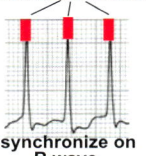

Pad/paddle placement for
synchronized cardioversion

synchronize on
R wave

18

Pulseless Arrest — Asystole & PEA
(assess appropriateness of resuscitation attempts)

Continue CPR (minimize interruptions in CPR)
(Confirm asystole in more than one lead)
Intubate (verify ETT placement and secure tube)

↓

Start IV/IO
Epinephrine 1 mg IV/IO (repeat every 3 – 5 min) *OR*:
Vasopressin 40 U IV/IO (single dose only)

↓

Consider Atropine 1 mg IV/IO, repeat every 3 – 5 min, max 3 mg
Continue CPR Immediately x 5 Cycles (~ 2 minutes)

❖ —Consider & Treat Possible Causes

Hypoxia — Ventilation
Hypovolemia — IV Fluids
Hypothermia — Warm patient
Hypokalemia — Restore electrolyte balance
Hypoglycemia — Dextrose
Hypothermia — Warm patient
Toxins — **Detoxify & appropriate therapies**
Coronary or Pulmonary Thrombosis — **Thrombolysis**
Trauma — Surgery / Control Hemorrhage
Cardiac Tamponade — Pericardiocentesis
Tension Pneumothorax — Thoracic Decompression
Hyperkalemia — **Sodium Bicarbonate 1 mEq/kg IV**
Metabolic Acidosis — ▼**Sodium Bicarbonate 1 mEq/kg IV**
Respiratory Acidosis — **Ventilation**

If VF/VT —see Pulseless Arrest V-Fib & V-Tach

↓

If pulse present: Assess vital signs, support airway & breathing, and give meds appropriate for BP, HR and ECG.

↓

If Asystole — Consider termination of efforts
(after successful intubation and medications, and no reversible causes are identified. Consider interval since arrest.)
▼**See Special Footnotes,** page 16

Bradycardia

(HR < 60 / minute with serious signs or symptoms: cx pain, dyspnea, ↓LOC, ↓BP, shock, pulmonary congestion, CHF, AMI)

Assess ABCs, Maintain airway, Give O$_2$, Start IV
Attach ECG, pulse oximeter, and BP cuff.
Assess vital signs, Get patient's history
Perform physical examination
↓

For Poor Perfusion
Transcutaneous Pacing for Mobitz II or 3rd° Block
Verify patient's capture and perfusion;
Use sedation as needed

Consider **Atropine 0.5 mg IV** ▼ q̄ 3 – 5 min, max: 3 mg
Consider **Epinephrine 2 – 10 mcg per minute, or:**
Dopamine 2 – 10 mcg/kg per minute
↓

Prepare for transvenous pacer
↓

For Pulseless Arrest —*See Pulseless Arrest Algorithm, page 19*

❖**Consider & Treat Causes, page 19**

Unsymptomatic Bradycardia
— *NOT* Type II (Mobitz) 2nd° or 3rd° AV heart block

Observe

▼**Do not delay TCP while starting IV, or waiting for atropine to work if patient is symptomatic.**
Atropine may not work for Mobitz (Type II) AV Block or 3rd° AV Block w/ IVR. Transplanted hearts may not respond to atropine — Begin pacing, & / or catecholamine infusion.

Tachycardias

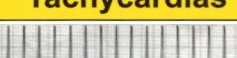

**Assess ABCs, Secure airway, Give O₂, Start IV, ECG,
Oximeter, SBP, Obtain history, examination; Get 12-lead ECG**
Consider & Treat Causes

Is Patient unstable, with serious signs or symptoms?

(S/Sx must be related to the tachycardia: chest pain, dyspnea,
↓LOC, ↓SBP, shock, pulmonary congestion, CHF, AMI.)

⚡ Immediate Synchronized Cardioversion — *See page 18*
(sedation if possible, but do not delay cardioversion)

For Pulseless Arrest — *See Pulseless Arrest Algorithm,* page 19

Stable Narrow Complex Tachycardia?

(obtain expert consultation when possible)

Regular?	Irregular?

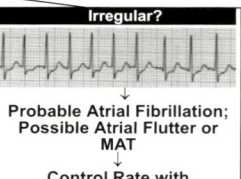

Regular?

↓

Vagal maneuvers *

**Adenosine 6 mg rapid IVP
Adenosine 12 mg, rapid IVP**
(may repeat once in 1 – 2 min)

If Rhythm Converts,
likely Reentry SVT

Treat Recurrence with
Adenosine, or:
• Diltiazem, • Beta-Blocker
If Rhythm Does NOT Convert,
likely A-Flutter, Ectopic AT,
or Ectopic JT

Control Rate with
• Diltiazem, • Beta-Blocker
Treat Underlying Causes.

Irregular?

↓

Probable Atrial Fibrillation;
Possible Atrial Flutter or
MAT

↓

Control Rate with
• Diltiazem, • Beta-Blocker

Continued Below

Wide-QRS Tachycardia of Uncertain Type:
(try to make a specific rhythm diagnosis with 12-lead ECG)

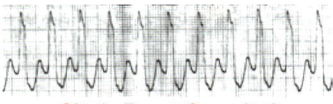

Obtain Expert Consultation

Regular?

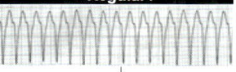

For VT or Uncertain
Rhythm
**Amiodarone 150 mg IV over
10 minutes**
May repeat, (Max dose:
2.2 gm IV / 24 hours)

↗ **Sync. cardioversion**
—*See* Cardioversion,
page 18

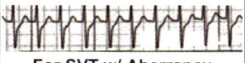

For SVT w/ Aberrancy

**Adenosine 6 mg rapid IVP
Adenosine 12 mg, rapid IVP**
(may repeat once in 1 – 2
min)

Irregular?

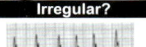

For Atrial Fibrillation w/
Aberrancy

Control Rate with
• **Diltiazem,** • **Beta-Blocker**

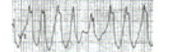

For Pre-excited Atrial Fib
(WPW)

**Consider Amiodarone 150
mg IV over 10 minutes**
(avoid adenosine, digoxin,
diltiazem, verapamil)

For Torsades de Pointes

**Magnesium 1 – 2 Gm IV
over 5 – 60 minutes,
followed by infusion**

*** CSM is contraindicated in patients with carotid bruits. Avoid ice
water immersion if pt. has ischemic heart disease.**

ACLS

Hypothermia

- **Remove wet clothing and Stop heat loss** (cover with blankets and insulating equipment)
- **Keep patient horizontal**
- **Move patient gently if possible, do not jostle**
- **Monitor core temperature and cardiac rhythm** (ECG may require needle electrodes through the skin)
- **Check responsiveness, breathing, pulse**

If Pulse & Breathing

34°C–36°C (mild hypothermia)
Passive rewarming

30°C–34°C (moderate hypothermia)
Passive rewarming
Active external rewarming of truncal areas only* (may use electric or charcoal warming devices, hot water bottles, heating pads, radiant heat sources, and warming beds)

<30°C (severe hypothermia)
Active internal rewarming sequence*

**Warm IV fluids (43°C)
Warm, humid O₂
(42°C–46°C)
Peritoneal lavage (KCl-free)
Extracorporeal rewarming
Esophageal rewarming tubes**

Continue rewarming until:
Core temperature > 35°C, *OR:*
Spontaneous Circulation, *OR:*
Resuscitation efforts cease

No Pulse / Apneic

**Start CPR
Defibrillate VF/VT x 1
Biphasic: 120 – 200J** *OR:*
**Monophasic 360 J
Resume CPR Immediately
Intubate, Ventilate with warm,
humid oxygen (42°– 46°C)*
Start IV, Administer warm
normal saline (43°C)***

Is core temperature < 30°C?

**Continue CPR
Withhold IV medications
Limit shocks for VF/VT to 1
Transport to ED**

Is core temperature ≥ 30°C?

**Continue CPR
Give IV meds as indicated** (longer than standard intervals)
Repeat defibrillation for VF/VT as core temperature rises
Start Active internal rewarming sequence* (left)

***Many experts think these should be done only in-hospital.**

Hypotension, Shock

Assess ABCs, Secure airway (verify placement, secure tube)
Administer oxygen, Start IV
Attach ECG monitor, pulse oximeter, automatic SBP
Assess vital signs, Review history
Perform physical examination
Get 12 lead ECG, portable chest X-Ray

What is the Most Likely Problem?

Volume problem? | *Rate problem?* | *Pump problem?*

Volume problem?
Administer:
IV Fluids
Blood transfusions
Cause-specific interventions
Consider vasopressors

Rate problem?
(Brady: page 20)
(Tachy: page 21)

Pump problem?
What is the BP?
(if possible, use invasive hemodynamic monitoring)

BP <70? 70–100? >100?

Systolic BP < 70 mm Hg:
Norepinephrine 0.5–30 mcg/min IV

Systolic BP 70–100 w/Shock:
Dopamine 2–20 mcg/kg/min*

Systolic BP 70–100 mm Hg without shock symptoms:
Dobutamine 2–20 mcg/kg/min*

Systolic BP >100 mm Hg:
Nitroglycerin 10–20 mcg/min

*Consider further actions especially if the patient has APE

[continue below]

Further considerations:
•**Treat reversible causes**
•**Pulmonary artery catheter**
•**Intra-aortic balloon pump**
•**Angiography & PCI**
•**Additional diagnostic studies**
•**Surgical interventions**
•**Additional drug therapy**

24

Acute Pulmonary Edema

Rate problem?

Too slow —*See* Bradycardia Algorithm, page 20
Too fast —*See* Tachycardia Algorithm, page 21

First-line actions:
Oxygen / Intubate p.r.n.
Nitroglycerin 0.4 mg SL
Furosemide 0.5 – 1 mg/kg IV
Morphine 2 – 4 mg IV

Second-line actions:
Nitroglycerin / Nitroprusside IV (if SBP >100 mm Hg)
Dopamine (if SBP 70 – 100 mm Hg **with** shock symptoms)
Dobutamine (if SBP >100 mm Hg, **no** shock symptoms)

Also Consider:
Treat reversible causes
Pulmonary artery catheter
Intra-aortic balloon pump
Angiography & PCI
Additional diagnostic studies
Surgical interventions
Additional drug therapy

STEMI Fibrinolytic Protocol
"Time is muscle"

"Door-to-Drug" time should be < 30 minutes.

- **S/S–Cx pain >15 min, but < 12hrs, not relieved by NTG.**
- **ECG & other findings consistent c̄ AMI.**
- **Cardiac risk factors? Hx? CAOx4?**
- **Age >35 yrs (>40 if female)?**
- **Give: O₂, NTG, MS, ASA** (if no contraindications)
- **Start 2 IVs,** (but don't delay transport)
- **Get Stat 12-lead ECG.** (Must show ST elevation, or new LBBB.)
- **Systolic/diastolic BP: R arm___/___ L arm___/___**
- **Complete Fibrinolytic Checklist: (all should be "No")**
- ☐ **Systolic BP >180 mm Hg**
- ☐ **Diastolic BP >110**
- ☐ **R arm vs L arm BP difference >15 mm Hg**
- ☐ **Hx Structural CNS Disease**
- ☐ **Head / Facial Trauma w/in 3 months**
- ☐ **Major trauma, surgery GI bleed w/in 6 weeks**
- ☐ **On blood thinners; bleeding/clotting problems**
- ☐ **Pregnancy**
- ☐ **CPR >10 minutes**
- ☐ **Advanced cancer, severe liver / renal disease**

Risk Profile / Indications for Transfer:

(if any are checked, consider transport to a hospital capable of angiography, PCI, and revascularization)
- ☐ **Heart rate ≥ 100 bpm and SBP ≤ 100 mm Hg, or**
- ☐ **Pulmonary edema (rales), or**
- ☐ **Signs of shock**
- ☐ **Contraindications to fibrinolytics**

• *If no contraindications and Dx of AMI is confirmed:*

Administer fibrinolytic. Also consider: **antiarrhythmics, anticoagulants,** and **standard MI treatments.** *Signs of reperfusion include:* pain relief, ST-segment normalization, reperfusion arrhythmias, resolution of conduction block, early CPK peak.

26

Ischemic Chest Pain Algorithm

1 Chest Pain Suggestive of Ischemia
↓

2 EMS Assessment
- ABCs, prepare for CPR; have defibrillator ready
- Give oxygen, aspirin, NTG, morphine as indicated
- **Oxygen** at 4 L/min; keep O_2 sat $\geq$ 90%
- **Aspirin** 160 – 325 mg
- **Nitroglycerin** SL, spray, or IV
- **Morphine** IV if pain not relieved with NTG
- Obtain 12-Lead ECG; if STEMI begin fibronolytic checklist
- Notify hospital to mobilze resources for STEMI
↓

3 Immediate ED Assessment & Treatment:
- Vitals, O2 sat, • Obtain IV access • Continue MONA
- Review 12-lead ECG
- Brief, targeted H & P; fibrinolytic checklist, especially contraindications
- Get initial serum cardiac marker levels
- Evaluate initial electrolyte and coagulation studies
- Portable chest x-ray (< 30 minutes)
↓

4 12-lead ECG Results:

5 ST elevation or new or presumably new LBBB: strongly suspicious for injury	**9** ST depression or T-wave inversion: strongly suspicious for ischemia	**13** Nondiagnostic ECG; no change in ST seg., or T waves
ST-elevation AMI	High-risk unstable angina / non-ST-elevation AMI	Intermediate / low-risk unstable angina
↓	↓	↓
6 Start adjunctive treatments (as indicated; no reperfusion delay) ✓ Beta-blockers ✓ Clopidogrel ✓ Heparin IV	**10** Start adjunctive treatments (as indicated; no contraindications) ✓ Nitroglycerin ✓ Beta-blockers ✓ Clopidogrel ✓ Heparin (UFH/LMWH) ✓ Glycoprotein IIb/IIIa inhibitor	**14** Develops high or intermediate risk? or Troponin
		No ↓
		15 Admit to ED: follow: ✓ Serial cardiac markers ✓ Serial/continuous ECGs ✓ ST seg. monitoring ✓ Consider stress test

↓ *Continued below*   ↓   ↓

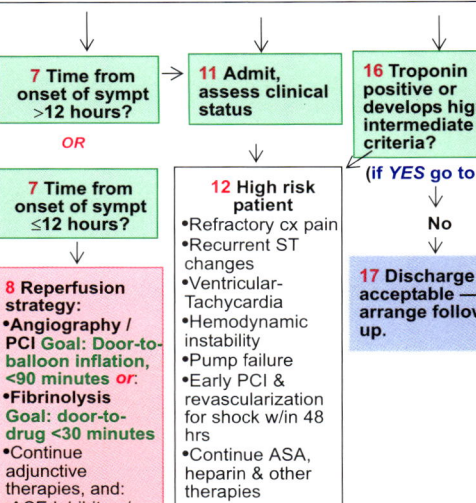

7 Time from onset of sympt >12 hours?

OR

7 Time from onset of sympt ≤12 hours?

8 Reperfusion strategy:
• Angiography / PCI Goal: Door-to-balloon inflation, <90 minutes *or*:
• Fibrinolysis Goal: door-to-drug <30 minutes
• Continue adjunctive therapies, and:
• ACE Inhibitors/ARB blockers within 24 hrs of onset S/Sx
• Statin therapy

11 Admit, assess clinical status

12 High risk patient
• Refractory cx pain
• Recurrent ST changes
• Ventricular-Tachycardia
• Hemodynamic instability
• Pump failure
• Early PCI & revascularization for shock w/in 48 hrs
• Continue ASA, heparin & other therapies
• ACE/ARB inhibitor
• Statin therapy

NOT high risk?
Risk-stratify by cardiology

16 Troponin positive or develops high or intermediate risk criteria?

(if *YES* go to 12)

No

17 Discharge acceptable — arrange follow-up.

(This algorithm provides general guidelines that may not apply to all patients. For all treatments, carefully consider the presence of proper indications and the absence of contraindications.)

3 Lead & MCL₁ Electrode Placement

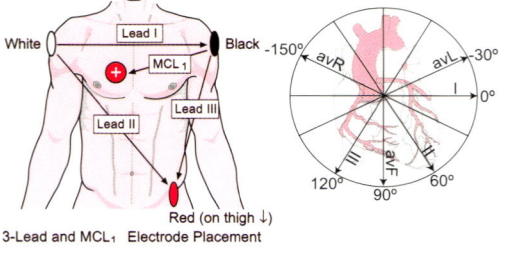

3-Lead and MCL₁ Electrode Placement

12 Lead Electrode Placement

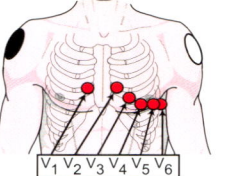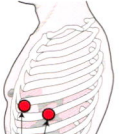

V₁: 4th interspace, just to the right of the sternum
V₂: 4th interspace, just to the left of the sternum
V₃: halfway between V₂ & V₄
V₄: 5th intercostal space, midclavicular line
V₅: anterior-axillary line, horizontal with V₄.
V₆: mid-axillary line, horizontal with V₄.
MCL₁: red lead on V₁, black lead on L arm–monitor L III.
MCL₆: red lead on V₆, black lead on R arm–monitor L I.
MC₄R: red lead on 5th ICS R mid-clavicular line, black lead on L arm – monitor L III.

Basic EKG Interpretation

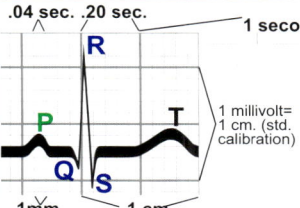

.04 sec. .20 sec.

1 second

R

P

Q S

T

1 millivolt=
1 cm. (std.
calibration)

1mm

1 cm

ECG waves:
P Wave: atrial depolarization
QRS Complex: ventricular depolarization
T Wave: ventricular repolarization

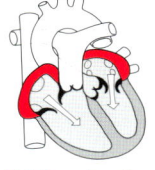

Atrial contraction

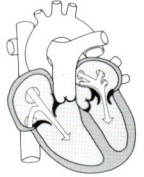

Ventricular contraction

Ventricular relaxation & passive filling

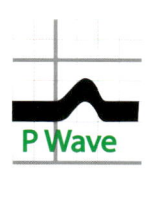

P Wave

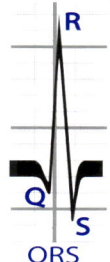

R

Q

S

QRS

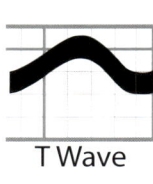

T Wave

30

Rapid Interpretation—12-Lead ECG

1 **Identify the rhythm.** If supraventricular (Sinus Rhythm, Atrial Fibrillation, Atrial Tachycardia, Atrial Flutter):

2 **Rule out LBBB** (QRS >120mS; & R,R' in I, or V_5, or V_6). LBBB confounds the Dx of AMI/ACS, (unless it is new-onset LBBB.)

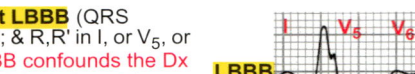

3 If no LBBB, **check for** ST segment elevation, **or** ST depression w/ T wave inversion, **or** pathologic Q waves.

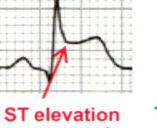
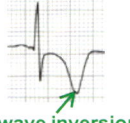
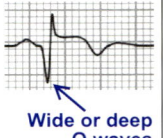

4 **ST elevation means acute MI**

T wave inversion may mean myocardial ischemia, or impending MI.

Wide or deep Q waves mean infarct.

4 **Rule out other confounders:** WPW (mimics infarct, BBB), pericarditis (mimics MI), digoxin (depresses STs), LVH (depresses STs, inverts T).

5 **Identify location of infarct & consider appropriate treatments** (MONA, PCI [or fibrinolytic], nitrate infusion, heparin, GP IIb, IIIa inhibitor, beta-blockers, antiarrhythmic, etc.).

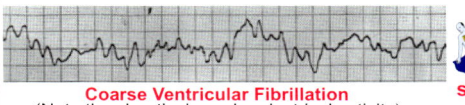

Coarse Ventricular Fibrillation
(Note the chaotic, irregular electrical activity)

shock

Fine Ventricular Fibrillation
(Note the low-amplitude, irregular electrical activity)

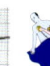
shock

Ventricular Tachycardia
(Note the rapid, wide complexes)

**shock
if no pulse**

Asystole
(Note the absence of electrical activity)

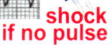
CPR

Pulseless Electrical Activity (PEA)
(Any organized EKG rhythm with no pulse)

CPR

32

Other Common EKG Rhythms

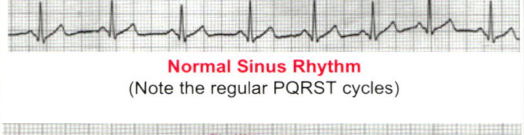

Normal Sinus Rhythm
(Note the regular PQRST cycles)

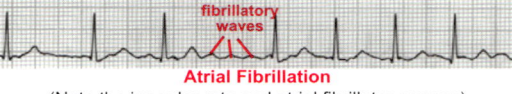

Atrial Fibrillation
(Note the irregular rate and atrial fibrillatory waves)

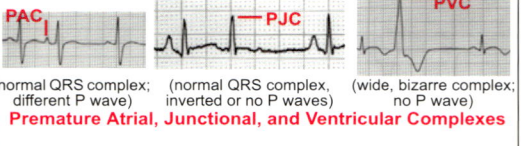

(normal QRS complex;   (normal QRS complex,   (wide, bizarre complex;
different P wave)   inverted or no P waves)   no P wave)

Premature Atrial, Junctional, and Ventricular Complexes

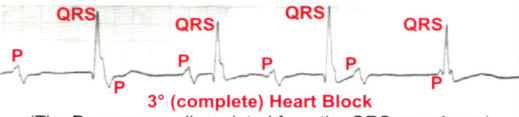

3° (complete) Heart Block
(The P waves are dissociated from the QRS complexes)

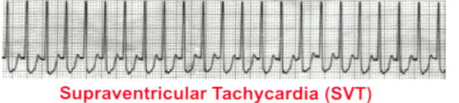

Supraventricular Tachycardia (SVT)
(Note the rapid, narrow QRS complexes)

Other Common EKG Rhythms

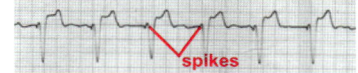

Electronic Ventricular Pacemaker
(Note the pacer spikes before each QRS)

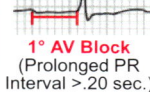

1° AV Block
(Prolonged PR
Interval >.20 sec.)

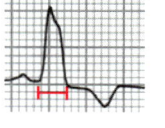 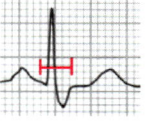

Bundle Branch Block
(Wide QRS >.12 sec)

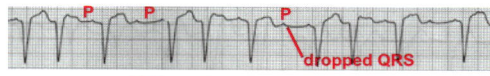

2° Heart Block, Wenckebach
(The PR interval lengthens, resulting in a dropped QRS)

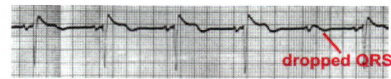

2° Heart Block, Mobitz
(The PR interval does not lengthen, but a QRS is dropped)

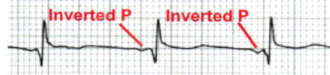

Junctional Rhythm
(Normal QRS complexes; inverted, or no P waves)

34

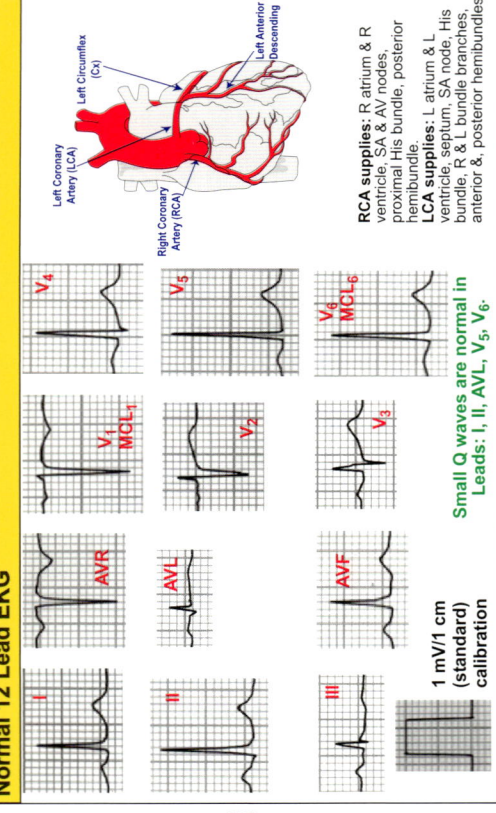

RCA supplies: R atrium & R ventricle, SA & AV nodes, proximal His bundle, posterior hemibundle.

LCA supplies: L atrium & L ventricle, septum, SA node, His bundle, R & L bundle branches, anterior &, posterior hemibundles.

Small Q waves are normal in Leads: I, II, AVL, V_5, V_6.

Left Coronary Artery (LCA)

Left Circumflex (Cx)

Left Anterior Descending

Right Coronary Artery (RCA)

V_4

V_5

V_6 MCL_6

V_1 MCL_1

V_2

V_3

AVR

AVL

AVF

I

II

III

1 mV/1 cm (standard) calibration

(If signs of AMI are not present on the initial ECG – perform serial ECGs)

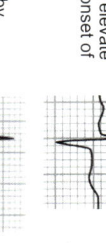

Injury
(ST segments usually elevate within minutes of the onset of cardiac chest pain)

Ischemia
(T waves invert fully by 24 hours)

Acute Infarction
(pathologic Q waves ≥ .03 sec or 1/3 height of QRS begin to form in 1 hour)

Old Infarction
(ST segments are normal; Q waves remain forever)

Reciprocal ST Depression
(found in leads away from the infarction)

Non-Q-Wave Infarction
(flat, depressed ST segments in two or more contiguous leads; or may have inverted T waves)

Early reperfusion in the definitive treatment for most AMI patients. The patient can lose 1% of salvageable myocardium for each minute of delay. Remember: *"Time is Muscle"*

36

Acute Anterior MI

(ST segment elevation ≥ 0.5 – 1 mm, with or without Q waves In two or more contiguous Leads $V_1–V_4$. Poor R wave progression* and inverted T waves may also be present. Reciprocal ST depression may be present in: II, III, AVF).

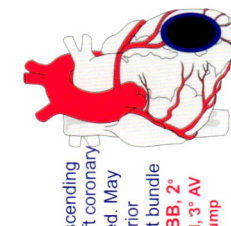

The anterior descending branch of the left coronary artery is occluded. May cause: Left anterior hemiblock; Right bundle branch block; **BBB, 2°** **AV block Mobitz II, 3° AV block with IVR, pump failure.**

3° block

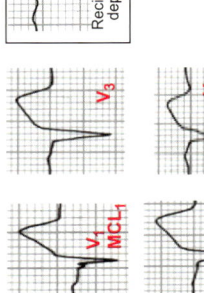

II
III
AVF
Reciprocal ST depression

V_3

V_4

V_1
MCL_1

V_2

*Note: LVH also can cause poor R wave progression & Q waves in $V_1 – V_2$. Rule it out first.

Acute Inferior MI

(ST segment elevation ≥ 0.5 – 1 mm in two or more contiguous Leads: II, III, AVF. Q waves and inverted T waves may also be present. Reciprocal ST depression may be present in Leads: I, AVL, $V_2 – V_4$.)

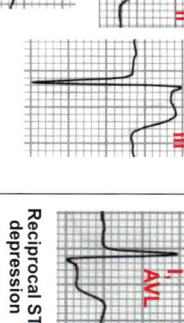

II

III

AVF

Reciprocal ST depression

I, AVL

V_2, V_3, V_4

Right Ventricle AMI accompanies Inferior AMI 30% of the time. Check Lead V_4R for elevated ST segment & Q wave.

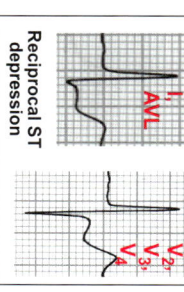

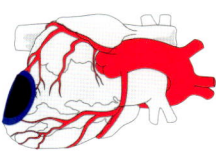

3° block δ IJR

II

The right (or left) coronary artery is occluded. May cause: Left posterior hemiblock; left axis deviation, ↓ BP, sinus bradycardia, 1° AV block, 2° AV block Mobitz I (Wenckenbach), 3° AV **block with IJR**

Acute Right Ventricle MI

(ST segment elevation in Lead: V_4R (MC_4R). Q wave and inverted T wave may also be present) Accompanies Inferior MI in 30% of cases.

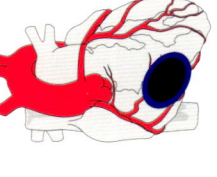

RCA is occluded. May cause: **AV block**, A-Fib, A-Flutter, right heart failure, JVD with clear lungs. **BP may drop if preload is reduced** (be cautious with morphine, NTG, furosemide). Treat hypotension with IV fluids, pacing.

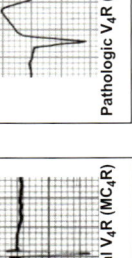

Normal V_4R (MC_4R)

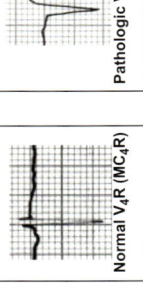

Pathologic V_4R (MC_4R)

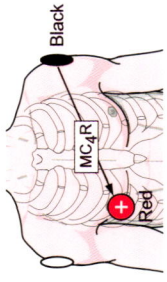

Black

Red

MC_4R

MC_4R Lead Placement: 5th interspace, right mid-clavicular line; monitor L III

(ST segment elevation ≥ 0.5 – 1 mm in Leads: I, AVL, V₅, V₆. Q waves and inverted T waves may also be present)

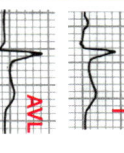
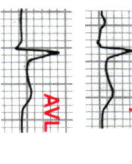

V₆, MCL₆

V₅

AVL

I

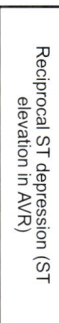

Reciprocal ST depression (ST elevation in AVR)

III, AVF

AVR

Note: Lateral MI May be a component of a multiple site infarction, including anterior, inferior and / or posterior MI.

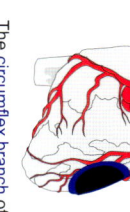

The circumflex branch of the left coronary artery is occluded. May cause: LV dysfunction, AV nodal block.

Acute Posterior MI*

(ST segment depression with or without large R waves in Leads: V_1, V_2, V_3. Inverted T waves may also be present)

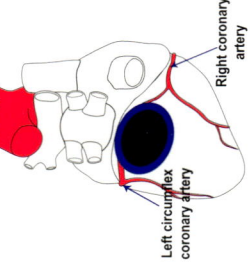

Right coronary artery

Left circumflex coronary artery

The right coronary artery or the circumflex branch of the left coronary artery is occluded. May cause: Sinus arrest.

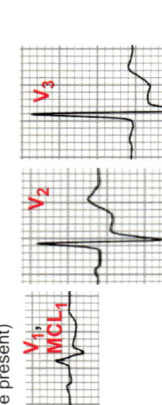

V_1, MCL$_1$

V_2

V_3

* Acute posterior MI is rarely seen alone. It is usually a component of a multiple site infarction, including inferior MI.

Note: RVH can also cause a large R wave in V_1. Rule out RVH first.

II

Sinus Arrest

Bundle Branch Block

(QRS ≥ .12 second)

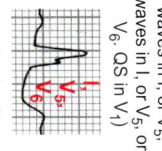

Left BBB
(Notched/slurred R waves in I, or V₅, or V₆. QS in V₁)

V₁, MCL₁

I, V₅, V₆

Note: if LBBB is Present, do not attempt to diagnose AMI using only EKG criteria.

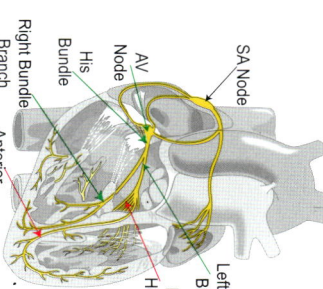

SA Node

AV Node

His Bundle

Right Bundle Branch

Left Bundle Branch

Posterior Hemibundle

Anterior Hemibundle

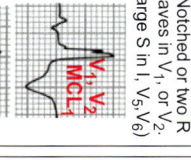

Right BBB
(Notched or two R waves in V₁, or V₂. Large S in I, V₅,V₆)

V₁, V₂, MCL₁

V₁, V₂, MCL₁

I, V₅, V₆

ACLS

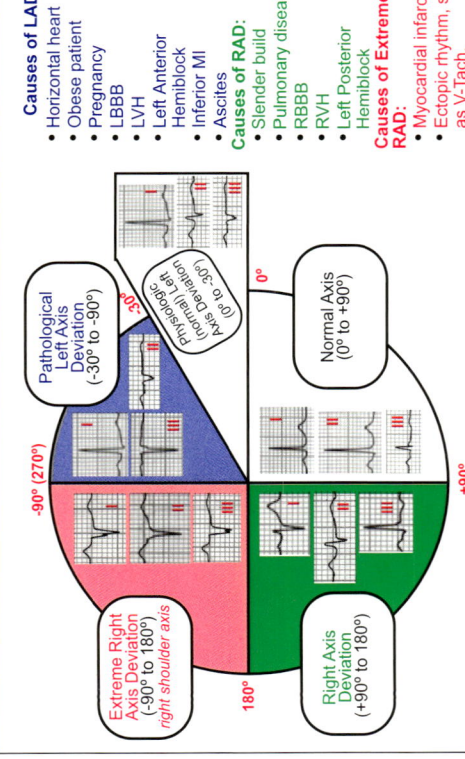

Causes of LAD:
- Horizontal heart
- Obese patient
- Pregnancy
- LBBB
- LVH
- Left Anterior Hemiblock
- Inferior MI
- Ascites

Causes of RAD:
- Slender build
- Pulmonary disease
- RBBB
- RVH
- Left Posterior Hemiblock

Causes of Extreme RAD:
- Myocardial infarction
- Ectopic rhythm, such as V-Tach.

Normal Axis (0° to +90°)

Physiologic Left Axis Deviation (0° to -30°)

Pathological Left Axis Deviation (-30° to -90°)

Extreme Right Axis Deviation (-90° to 180°) right shoulder axis

Right Axis Deviation (+90° to 180°)

0°

+90°

180°

-30°

-90° (270°)

Wide Complex Tachycardia

(V-Tach vs. SVT with aberrancy)

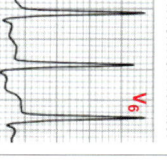

V-Tach

V6
MCL6

V1

V1

Consider lidocaine

Suggestive EKG signs for V-Tach:

☐ Fusion beats: diagnostic
☐ Capture beats: diagnostic
☐ Extreme RAD (-90° to 180°)
☐ QRS > 0.14 sec.
☐ QRS V1 – V6 are all negative or all positive
☐ L rabbit ear > R rabbit ear in V1
☐ Wide initial R wave in V1
☐ A-V dissociation (independent P waves)
☐ Small R wave in V6, or QS in V6
☐ Hx: MI, LVH, CAD, cardiomyopathy

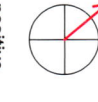

Suggestive EKG signs for SVT:

☐ Irregular rhythm: consider A-Fib
☐ Associated P waves: consider PSVT

When in doubt, treat for V-Tach*

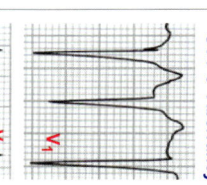

SVT c̄ Aberrancy

V6

V1

Consider adenosine

Electrolyte / Drug Effects

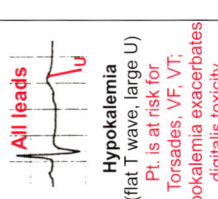

tall; peaked T

Hyperkalemia

(Tall, peaked T waves; wide QRS and loss of P waves in extreme cases)

Pt. is at risk for asystole, VF.

All leads

u

Hypokalemia

(flat T wave, large U)

Pt. is at risk for Torsades, VF, VT; hypokalemia exacerbates digitalis toxicity

Digitalis Effect

(Depressed ST segments; asymmetrically inverted T)

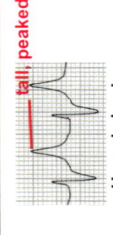

Torsades de Pointes (2° anything that prolongs the QT interval: bradycardia, digitalis toxicity, quinidine, procainamide, disopyramide, phenothiazines, hypokalemia, hypomagnesemia, hypocalcemia, insecticide poisoning, subarachnoid hemorrhage, TCA OD)

ST Segment Elevation– Benign Normal Variant
(upsloping, mildly elevated ST segments in a few leads; no reciprocal ST depression)

depressed PR Segment   elevated ST segment & T wave

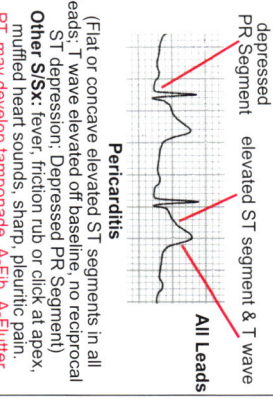

Pericarditis
(Flat or concave elevated ST segments in all leads; T wave elevated off baseline, no reciprocal ST depression; Depressed PR Segment)

Other S/Sx: fever, friction rub or click at apex, muffled heart sounds, sharp, pleuritic pain.
PT. may develop tamponade, A-Fib, A-Flutter, PAT

All Leads

COPD (small QRSs in limb leads) RVH may also be present.

I, II, III, AVR, L, F

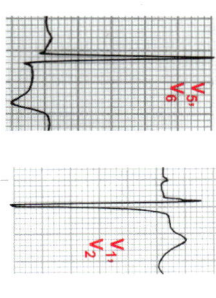

Left Ventricular Hypertrophy
(R waves ≥ 25mm in V_5, V_6; or S waves ≥ 25mm in V_1, V_2)

V_5, V_6

V_1, V_2

WPW & LGL Syndromes

Wolff-Parkinson-White Syndrome
(short PR, wide QRS, delta wave) **Patient is prone to PSVT.**

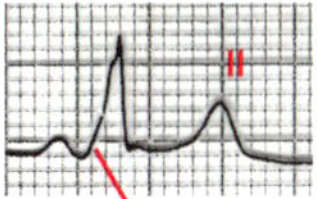

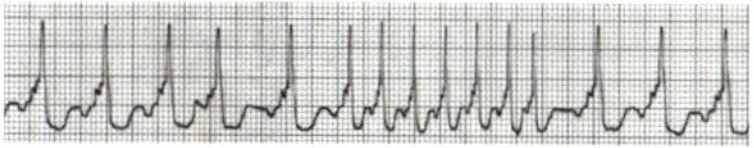

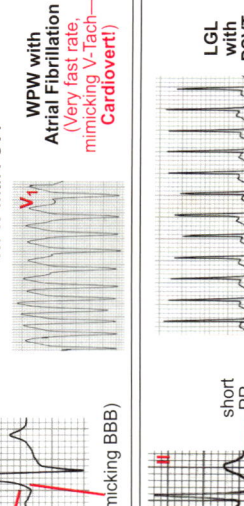

WPW with PSVT

WPW with Atrial Fibrillation
(Very fast rate, mimicking V-Tach—**Cardiovert!**)

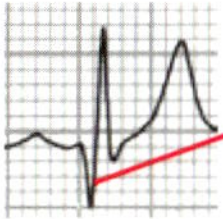

V₁

LGL with PSVT

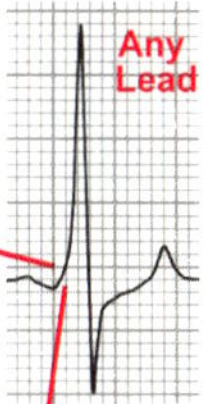

Any Lead

(mimicking BBB)

WPW (mimicking a Q wave)

II

delta wave

Lown-Ganong-Levine Syndrome
(short PR, normal QRS width) **Patient is prone to PSVT and V-Tach.**

short PR

II

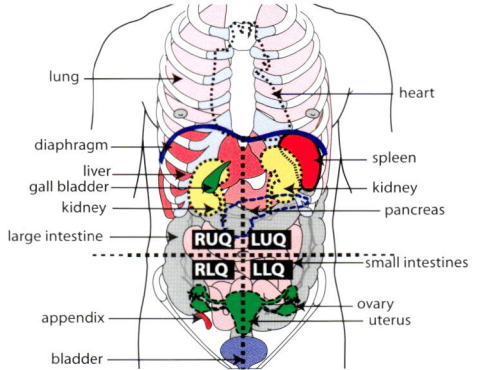

Common Causes of Abdominal Pain

- **Epigastric:** AMI, gastroenteritis, ulcer, esophageal disease, heartburn.
- **RUQ:** gall stones, hepatitis, liver disease, pancreatitis, appendicitis, perforated duodenal ulcer, AMI, pneumonia.
- **LUQ:** gastritis, pancreatitis, AMI, pneumonia.
- **LLQ:** ruptured ectopic pregnancy, ovarian cyst, PID, kidney stones, diverticulitis, enteritis, abdominal abscess.
- **RLQ:** appendicitis, ruptured ectopic pregnancy, enteritis, diverticulitis, PID, ovarian cyst, kidney stones, abdominal abscess, strangulated hernia.
- **Midline:** bladder infection, aortic aneurysm, uterine disease, intestinal disease, early appendicitis.
- **Diffuse Pain:** pancreatitis, peritonitis, appendicitis, gastroenteritis, dissecting / rupturing aortic aneurysm, diabetes, ischemic bowel, sickle cell crisis.

Abdominal Pain

HX—Ask PAIN QUESTIONS & GENERAL HISTORY.
N&V? (color / quality of emesis) bowel movements, dysuria, menstrual Hx, fv, postural hypotension, referred shoulder pain? Is pt. pregnant? Which trimester? Consider ectopic pregnancy. Genitourinary, vaginal or rectal bleeding / discharge? Examine all 4 quadrants: abdominal tenderness, guarding, rigidity, bowel tones present? Distension, pulsatile mass? Record recent intake and GI habits. Vitals (sitting & supine), chemstrip. Peripheral pulses equal?

✚—Position of comfort and NPO. Consider pulse oximetry. O_2, IV (adjusted to vitals), consider EKG for epigastric pain.

Caution—Consider aortic aneurysm; ectopic pregnancy, DKA. **Epigastric abdominal pain may be cardiac.**

▼Abdominal Aortic Aneurysm: severe abdominal pain, pulsatile mass, hypotension.

▼Acute MI: chest "pressure" or epigastric pain radiating to L arm or jaw; diaphoresis, N&V, SOB, pallor, dysrhythmias.

▼Appendicitis: N&V, RLQ or periumbilical pain, fv, shock.

▼Bowel Obstruction: N&V (fecal odor), localized pain.

▼Cholecystitis: acute onset RUQ pain & tenderness (may be referred to R shoulder / scapula)—may be related to high fat meal; N&V, anorexia, fever. "Female, fat, 40".

▼Ectopic Pregnancy: missed period, pelvic pain, abnormal vaginal bleeding, dizziness.

▼Food Poisoning: N&V, diffuse abdominal pain and cramping, diarrhea, fever, weakness, dizziness. Severe symptoms: descending paralysis, respiratory compromise.

▼Hepatic Failure: jaundice, confusion/coma, edema, bleeding and bruising, renal failure, fever, anorexia, dehydration.

▼Kidney Stone: constant or colicky severe flank pain, extreme restlessness, hematuria, N&V.

▼Pancreatitis: severe, "sharp" or "twisting" epigastric or LUQ pain radiating to back; N&V, diaphoresis, abdominal distention, signs of shock, fever.

▼Ulcer: "burning", epigastric pain, N&V, possible hematemesis, hypotension, decreased bowel sounds.

Abuse—Child, Domestic, Elder

Remove patient from the environment; Transport to hospital; Report possible abuse to police, ED staff, and Child Welfare office. Call for police assistance if needed to remove pt. from the scene. **Don't confront the alleged abuser.** Document your findings, any statements made by child, parent, others. Provide medical care as needed. If sexual abuse, do not allow pt. to wash.

Child Abuse

HX—Any unusual MOI, or one that does not match the child's injury/ illness. Parents may accuse the child of hurting him/herself, or may be vague / contradictory in providing Hx. There may be a delay in seeking medical care. **The child may not cling to mother.** Fx in any child < 2 y.o.; **multiple injuries in various stages of healing,** or on many parts of the body; obvious cigarette burns / wire marks; **malnutrition;** insect infestation, chronic skin infection, unkempt pt.

Domestic Abuse HX

Repeated ED visits with injuries becoming more severe with each visit; **Minimizing the seriousness** or frequency of the injuries; Seeking treatment one or more days after the injury; **Injuries that are not likely to have been caused by the accident reported;** Overprotective significant other who does not allow the patient to be alone with the health care professional; **Fractures in different stages of healing** according to radiographic findings; History of child abuse to patient or partner.

Elder Abuse HX

Fractures or bruises at various stages of healing; Unexplained bruises or cigarette burns on the torso or extremities; Soft tissue injuries from signs of restraint use; Head injuries; Malnourishment, listlessness, dehydration unexplained; **Poor hygiene,** inappropriate clothing; Decubitus ulcer, **urine and feces on body and clothing;** Unusual interaction between caregiver and patient.

Airway Obstruction, See *Choking*, page 57

Allergic Reaction

HX—Mild reaction? (local swelling only); or serious systemic reaction? (hives, pallor, bronchospasm, wheezing, upper airway obstruction with stridor, swelling of throat, hypotension); **If cardiac arrest, treat per ACLS).**

▼If bee sting, remove stinger (scrape, don't squeeze it).
- For mild local reaction: wash area, apply cold pack.
- For serious reaction: secure airway, ventilate, O$_2$; *large bore IV, titrate to BP > 90; EKG; **Epinephrine: 1:1,000 SQ, (Adult: 0.3 – 0.5 cc); (Pediatric: 0.01 cc/kg; 0.3 cc max)**.*

CAUTION: Epinephrine may cause arrhythmias or angina.

Altered Mental Status

▼**Consider: CVA / TIA / Stroke, hypoglycemia, postictal, alcohol, drugs, hypovolemia, head injury, hypothermia, HazMat, sepsis, shock, cardiogenic, vasovagal.**

HX—Ask **PAIN QUESTIONS & GENERAL HISTORY**. Time of onset: slow or fast? **Seizure activity?** Was pt. sitting, standing, lying? Is pt. pregnant? (consider ectopic pregnancy). Any recent illness, or trauma? Current level of consciousness? Neurological status and psychological status? Any vomiting **(bloody or coffee-ground)? Melena (black tarry stool) Any signs of recent trauma?**

✚—**General treatment — Protect airway.** Give O$_2$ PRN, Be prepared to assist ventilations. *Monitor EKG, vitals.*

✚—**Cardiac: Support ABCs. Vitals, O$_2$, *treat per ACLS***

✚—**Coma: (If multiple patients, suspect toxins — protect yourself!)** Any odor at scene? — Consider HazMat. Were there any preceding symptoms or **H/A?** Past Hx: HTN, diabetes? Medications? Check scene for pill bottles or syringes and bring along. Get vitals, LOC & neuro findings, pupils; Any signs of trauma, drug abuse? Skin: color, temperature, rash, welts, facial or extremity asymmetry, Medic Alert™ tag?

WARNING: Ensure your safety, then safety of pt & others.

Secure airway, ventilate with 100% O_2, protect C-spine. Start IV. Get chemstrip. Consider glucose, naloxone. Monitor vital signs, O_2 saturation, & EKG.

Caution—Protect airway, suction as needed.

✚—**Sepsis / Infection:** O_2, IV, Vitals. IV fluids for hypotension.

✚—**Syncope:** Position of comfort, O_2, IV, Vitals, EKG. Consider IV fluids for hypotension.

Caution—Syncope in middle-aged or elderly patients is often cardiac. Occult internal bleeding may cause syncope.

Burns—(Also *see Burn Chart,* page 11)

HX—**Airway burns?** (soot in mouth, red mouth, singed nasal hairs, **cough, hoarseness, dyspnea**)? Was patient in enclosed space? How long? **Did patient lose consciousness?** Was there an explosion? Toxic fumes? Hx cardiac or lung disease? Estimate % of burns & depth. Other trauma? **Significant burns = blistered or charred areas, or burns of the hands, feet, face, airway, genitalia.**

✚—**Stop the burning—extinguish clothing if smouldering.**

- Remove clothing if not adhered to skin; remove jewelry.
- Vitals, give high flow O_2, assist ventilations if needed.

1st & 2nd degree burns: If < 20%, apply wet dressings.

Moderate to severe burns: cover with DSD &/or burn sheet. Leave blisters intact. Start large bore IV, treat for shock or % burn. Monitor EKG.

Chemical burns: Brush off any dry chemical then flush with copious amounts of water or saline. For lime: brush off excess, then flush;—For phosphorus: use alcohol or **copious** amounts of water.

(Con't next page)

Electrical burns: Apply DSD to entry and exit wounds. Start large bore IV, titrate for shock. Monitor EKG—treat dysrhythmias per ACLS.

Caution—Consider child abuse in pediatric patients. Do not apply ointments to burns. Avoid starting IV in burned area if possible.

Remember: burned firefighters may be having an AMI.

Childbirth—(Also *see OB/GYN Emerg.*, page 62)

HX—Timing of contractions? intensity? Does mother have urge to push or to move bowels? Has amniotic sac ruptured? Medications — any medical problems? Vital signs, Check for:

- **Vaginal bleeding** or amniotic fluid; note color of fluid
- **Crowning** (means imminent delivery)
- **Abnormal presentation:** foot, arm, breech, cord, shoulder.
- Transport immediately if patient has had previous C-section, known multiple births, any abnormal presentation, excessive bleeding, or if pregnancy is not full-term and child will be premature.
- ✚ **Normal**—control delivery using gloved hand to guide head, suction mouth & nose, deliver, keep infant level with perineum, clamp & cut cord 8"–10" from **infant, warm & dry infant,** stimulate infant by drying with towel, **make sure respirations are adequate. Normal VS are: Pulse: >120, Resp >40, BP 70, Weight 3.5 kg.**

Give baby to mother to nurse at breast. Get APGAR scores at 1 and 5 minutes after birth.

If excessive post-partum bleeding, treat for shock, massage uterus to aid contraction, have mother nurse infant, *start large bore IV*, transport without waiting for placenta to deliver. Bring it with you to the hospital. Get mother's vital signs.

Most births are normal — reassure mom & dad.

APGAR Scale

	0 points	1 point	2 points	1 Min.	5 Min.
Heart rate	**Absent**	**<100**	**>100**		
Resp. Effort	**Absent**	**Slow, irreg.**	**Strong cry**		
Muscle Tone	Flaccid	Some flex.	Act. Motion		
Irritability	No response	Some	Vigorous		
Color	Blue, pale	Body: pink Ext: Blue	Fully pink		
			TOTAL:		

Infants with scores of 7–10 usually only need supportive care. **A score of 4 – 6 indicates moderate depression. Infants with scores of 3 or less require aggressive resuscitation.**

❖**Breech:** Call OLMC. If head won't deliver, consider applying gentle pressure on mother's abdomen. If unsuccessful, insert two gloved fingers in vagina between baby's face and vaginal wall to create airway. **Rapid transport.**

❖**Cord Presents:** Call OLMC. Place mother in trendelenburg & knee-chest position, hold pressure on baby's head to relieve pressure on cord, check pulses in cord, keep cord moist with saline dressing, O_2, **rapid transport,** *start IV en route.*

❖**Foot / leg presentation:** Call OLMC. Support presenting part, place mother in trendelenburg & knee-chest position, O_2, **rapid transport,** *start IV en route.*

❖**Cord around neck: unwrap cord from neck** and deliver normally, keep face clear, suction mouth & nose, etc.

❖**Infant not breathing:** Stimulate with dry towel, rub back, flick soles of feet with finger. **Suction mouth and nose. Ventilate with BVM & 100% O_2** (this will revive most infants). **Begin chest compressions if HR <60.** Ventilate with 100% O_2. If child does not respond, contact OLMC & reassess ventilation, lung sounds (pneumothorax? obstruction?) O_2 connected? *Ventilate. Consider Intubation, IV fluids 10cc/kg, glucose 2cc/kg D25%W, Epinephrine 0.01 mg/kg IV/IO, or 0.1 mg/kg 1:1000 ET.*

Rapid transport. Failure to respond usually indicates hypoxia.

Chest Pain

Consider: AMI, CHF, APE, pneumothorax, pneumonia, bronchitis, pulmonary embolus.

HX—Ask **PAIN QUESTIONS & GENERAL HX. Syncope, dizziness, weakness, diaphoresis?** Fever, **pallor? Dyspnea?**

Past Hx: chest trauma? cardiac or respiratory problems, diabetes, high blood pressure, heart failure? **Lung sounds, JVD? Peripheral or pulmonary edema,** general appearance?

✚—Position of comfort, reassure patient, vitals, Give O_2, Monitor EKG, Start IV, Consider nitroglycerine for cardiac chest pain: 0.4 mg SL q̄ 5 minutes (max: 3 doses). Consider aspirin for AMI. **Notify ED if your cardiac patient is a possible fibrinolytic candidate, and transport ASAP.**

Caution—Treat dysrhythmias according to ACLS.

❖**Acute MI:** severe, crushing chest pain, or substernal "pressure", radiating to the left arm, or jaw. N&V, SOB, diaphoresis, pallor, dysrhythmias, HTN or hypotension.

❖**Aortic Dissection:** sudden onset "tearing" chest or back pain, tachycardia, HTN or hypotension, diaphoresis, possible unequal pulses or unequal BP in extremities.

❖**Cholecystitis:** acute onset RUQ pain & tenderness (may be referred to R shoulder / scapula)—may be related to high fat meal; N&V, anorexia, fever. "Female, fat, 40".

❖**Hiatal Hernia:** positional epigastric pain.

❖**Musculo-Skeletal:** pain on palpation, respiration; obvious signs of trauma.

❖**Pleurisy:** pain on inspiration, fever, pleural friction rub.

❖**Pneumonia:** fever, shaking, chills, pleuritic chest pain, crackles, productive cough, tachycardia, diaphoresis.

❖**Pulmonary Embolus:** sudden onset SOB, cough, chest pain which is sharp and pleuritic, tachycardia, rapid respirations, O_2 sat <94%, apprehension, diaphoresis, hemoptysis, crackles.

❖**Ulcer:** "burning" epigastric pain, N&V, possible hematemesis, hypotension, decreased bowel sounds.

CPR: Adult, Child, or Infant

1 **Determine unresponsiveness**
2 **Call for assistance** / have someone get defibrillator / AED
3 **Position patient supine** on hard, flat surface
4 **Open airway:** head-tilt/chin-lift
5 **Check breathing:** f none: ventilate x 2 (make chest rise)
6 **Check pulse;** if none: begin chest compressions, 30:2*; push hard & fast — minimize interruptions in CPR
7 **Attach AED to adult (& child >1 y.o.);** follow voice prompts
8 If shockable rhythm (VF or VT), shock x1
9 **Resume CPR immediately — do not interrupt CPR**!
10 **Recheck pulse** after 5 cycles of CPR; if no pulse
11 **Continue CPR** and go to Pulseless Cardiac Arrest on page 17
12 **Recheck pulse & rhythm after every 5 cycles of CPR

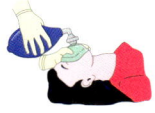

Start CPR & attach AED as soon as it arrives.

head-tilt / chin lift

nipple line ➡

CPR	Ratio	Rate	Depth	Check Pulse
Adult: 1 Person	30:2	100	1-1/2"–2"	Carotid
Adult: 2 Person	30:2	100	1-1/2"–2"	Carotid
Child: 1 Person	30:2	100	1/3–1/2 cx	Carotid
Child: 2 Person	15:2	100	1/3–1/2 cx	Carotid
Infant: 1 Person	15:2	100	1/3–1/2 cx	Brachial, Fem.
Newborn: 2 Pers	15:2	100	1/3–1/2 cx	Brachial, Fem.

56

Choking

For Responsive Choking Adult or Child

1 If patient can not talk or has stridor, or cyanosis:
2 **Perform Heimlich Maneuver;** (may also use back slaps—use chest thrusts if pt is pregnant or obese) repeat until successful or pt. is unconscious:
3 **Begin CPR / Call for assistance**
4 **Open airway; head tilt-chin lift (look and remove object if visible):**
5 Ventilate with two breaths—if unable:
6 **Reposition head**; attempt to ventilate—if unable:
7 **Perform chest compressions (30:2)**
8 **Repeat: inspect mouth → remove object → ventilate → chest compressions** until successful.
9 Consider **laryngoscopy** and removal of object by **forceps, ET intubation, transtracheal ventilation, cricothyrotomy.**
10 If pt. resumes breathing, place in the recovery position.

For Unresponsive Choking Adult or Child

1 **Determine unresponsiveness**
2 **Call for assistance**
3 **Position patient supine** on hard, flat surface
4 **Open airway** — head-tilt / chin-lift; (look and remove object if visible):
5 **Attempt to ventilate** — if unable:
6 **Reposition head & chin, attempt to ventilate** — if unable:
7 **Begin chest compressions 30:2**
8 **Repeat: inspect mouth → remove object → ventilate → chest compressions** until successful.
9 Consider **laryngoscopy and removal of object by forceps, ET intubation, transtracheal ventilation cricothyrotomy.**
10 If pt. resumes breathing, place in the recovery position.

For Choking Infant

1 **Confirm obstruction**: if infant can not make sounds, breathe, cry, or is cyanotic;
2 **Invert infant on arm**. Support head by cupping face in hand. **Perform 5 back blows & 5 chest thrusts** until object is expelled or pt becomes unconscious
3 **Repeat until successful**
4 **If pt becomes unconscious, start CPR**
5 **Open airway & ventilate x 2**; if unable;
6 **Reposition head & chin, attempt to ventilate again;**
7 Begin chest compressions 30:2.
8 **Repeat: inspect mouth → remove object → ventilate → chest compressions**
9 Consider **laryngoscopy** and removal of object by **forceps, ET intubation, transtracheal ventilation, cricothyrotomy**
10 **If pt. resumes breathing, place in the recovery position**.

Drowning and Near Drowning

HX—How long was patient submerged? Fresh or salt water? Cold water (<40°F)?
Diving accident? Immobilize spine.
S/S — Vitals, pulse oximetry, Neurological status, GCS, Crackles or pulmonary edema with respiratory distress?
✚—Open airway, suction, assist ventilations, start CPR. C-Spine: stabilize before removing patient from water. O_2, IV, Monitor EKG. If hypothermic: use heated O_2 & follow hypothermia protocols. Conserve heat with blankets.
Caution—All unconscious patients should have C-spine immobilization. All near-drowning patients should be transported. Many deteriorate later and develop pulmonary edema.
Prepare for vomiting; Intubate if unconscious.

58

Hyperglycemia

HX—Slow onset, excessive urination, thirst. When was insulin last taken? Abdominal cramps, N&V? Mental status, high glucose on chemstrip, skin signs, dehydration? Respirations: deep & rapid? Breath odor: acetone, fruity?

✚—Secure airway, get vital signs, give O$_2$, large bore IV fluid challenge (balanced salt solution). Monitor EKG.

Hypoglycemia / Insulin Shock

HX—Sudden onset, low blood glucose on Chemstrip. Last insulin dose? Last meal? Mental status? Diaphoresis, **H/A**, blurred vision, dizziness, tachycardia, tremors, seizures?

✚—Support ABCs, Give O$_2$, Take vitals, Start IV. Give 50cc D50%W if patient comatose (perform chemstrip $\overline{a}$ & $\overline{p}$). Do not give oral glucose if airway is compromised.

Caution— Hypoglycemia can mimic a stroke or intoxication. Seizures, coma, and confusion are common symptoms. **When in doubt about the diagnosis, give glucose IV or PO.**

HYPOGLYCEMIA VS. HYPERGLYCEMIA

Also known as	HYPOGLYCEMIA "Insulin Shock"	"HYPERGLYCEMIA DKA" "Ketoacidosis"
Incidence	More common	Less common
Blood sugar	Low (≤ 80 mg%)	High (≥ 180 mg%)
Onset	Rapid (minutes)	Gradual (days)
Skin	Moist, pale	Dry, warm
Respirations	Normal	Deep or Rapid
Pulse	Normal or fast	Rapid, weak
Breath odor	Normal	Acetone/Ketone odor
Seizures	Common	Uncommon
Dehydration	No	Yes
Urine output	Normal	Excessive
Thirst	Normal	Very Thirsty
Mental status	Disoriented, Coma	Awake, weak, tired
Treatment	Glucose IV or PO	IV Fluids, Insulin, K+
Recovery	Rapid (minutes)	Gradual (days)

When in doubt about the diagnosis, give glucose IV or PO.

Hyperthermia / Heat Stroke

HX—Onset? Exercise- or drug- (cocaine) induced? Vitals, temperature, Skin: warm, dry?

✚—Remove from hot environment. Secure airway. Give O_2. Undress and begin cooling patient. Consider cold packs to groin, armpits

Evaporation and convection measures work best (but avoid causing shivering as this may increase pts. temp.) *Start large bore IV. Consider fluid challenge. Monitor EKG. Reassess vital signs en route.*

Caution— Rapid cooling is key. **Don't delay transport**.

Hypothermia (*Also* see page 23)

HX—Vital signs, mental status. **Is patient cold? Shivering?** Evidence of local injury?

Mild hypothermia: shivering, ↑HR, ↑RR, lethargy, confusion.

Moderate hypothermia: ↓ respirations, ↓HR, rigidity, ↓L.O.C., "J wave" on EKG.

Severe hypothermia: coma, ↓BP, ↓HR, acidosis, VF, asystole.

✚—Secure airway. Remove patient from cold environment. Give heated O_2. A severely hypothermic patient may breathe slowly. Monitor EKG, large bore IV

If cardiac arrest: start CPR. Contact OLMC.

Cut wet clothing off (do not pull off) wrap patient with blankets. Record vital signs, including temperature.

Caution—Handle patient gently. Jostling can cause cardiac arrest. **If patient is not shivering, do not ambulate**. Stimulating the airway can cause cardiac arrest.

Infectious Diseases

Disease…	Spread by…	Risk to you…
AIDS / HIV	IV / Sex / Blood products	↓ Immune function, Pneumonias, Cancer
ANTHRAX	**Cutaneous:** contact with skin lesions	Infection = 25% mortality, but much lower if treated
	Ingestion: eating contaminated meat	Infection = high mortality, unless treated with antibiotics
	Pulmonary: inhaled spores	Infection = 95% mortality, but much lower if treated
Hepatitis A*	Fecal-oral	Acute hepatitis
Hepatitis B*	IV / Sex / Birth / Blood	Acute & chronic hepatitis, Cirrhosis, Liver CA
Hepatitis C	Blood	Chronic hepatitis, Cirrhosis, Liver CA
Hepatitis D	IV / Sex / Birth	Chronic liver disease
Hepatitis E	Fecal-oral	↑ Mortality to pregnant women and fetus
Herpes	Skin contact	Skin lesions, shingles
Meningitis*	Nasal secretions	Low risk to rescuer
Tuberculosis	Sputum / cough / IV / Body fluids	Active tuberculosis, pulmonary infection

Universal Precautions / BSI

✓ **Wear gloves for all patient contacts and for all contacts with body fluids.**
✓ **Wash hands after patient contact.**
✓ **Wear a mask for patients who are coughing or sneezing. Place a mask on the patient too.**
✓ **Wear eye shields or goggles when body fluids may splash.**
✓ **Wear gowns when needed.**
✓ **Wear utility gloves for cleaning equipment.**
✓ **Don't recap, cut, or bend needles.**
✓ ***Get vaccinated against Hepatitis A, B, and Meningitis A, C, W, Y.**

CAUTION: Report every exposure, get immediate treatment!

❖ **Abruptio Placenta:** Separation of placenta from uterine wall. Usually occurs > 20 weeks gestation. S/S: painful 3rd trimester vaginal bleeding (dark red); hypovolemic shock, hypotension, tachycardia, fetal distress ; ↓ FHT, ↑ fundal height, pale skin, diaphoresis. Give O$_2$, *start IV,* **Rapid transport.** Pt. may need C-section.

❖ **Placenta previa:** placenta covers cervical os, can occur during 2nd & 3rd trimester. S/S: painless bright red bleeding, possible hypotension, tachycardia; *start IV*, O$_2$, **Rapid transport.** Pt may require C-section.

❖ **Preeclampsia / PIH:** (pregnancy-induced hypertension) HTN, H/A, proteinuria, edema of hands, feet, face & sacrum, weight gain, ↓ urine output, visual disturbances, possible ↑ liver enzymes, ↑ neurologic reflexes, ↑ chances of seizures, ↓ FHT. Transport quietly & gently. Monitor vitals, *IV;* treat HTN with apresoline or mag sulfate; OB consult; supportive care; Seizure precautions: diazepam, phenytoin, calcium gluconate 10%.

Physiologic Changes During Pregnancy							
BP	Pulse	CO	ECG	Resp	ABG	Blood	Other
↓	↑	↑	T wave changes L II, avF, avL	↑Resp Rate ↑Tidal Vol. ↑Vital Capacity ↓Functional Residual Capacity	↑pH ↑PaO$_2$ ↓PaCO$_2$ ↓HCO$_3$ Resp. Alkalosis	↓HCT ↑WBC ↑Fibrinogen ↑Clot. Factors Prone to DIC ↑Blood Volume	↑N/V aspiration ↑Injury: uterus, pelvis, bladder ↑Falls ↑Peripheral venous pressure

Organ Donations

Tissue	Age	Restrictions
Bone	15-75	No IV drug use, no malignancy, no transmissible diseases
Eyes	Any age	No systemic infection, no IV drug use, no transmissible diseases
Heart valves	NB - 55	No IV drug use, no malignancy, no transmissible disease
Organs	NB- 70	Brain dead or potential to meet brain death, ventilator dependent
Skin	15-75	No IV drug use, no malignancy, no transmissible disease

There are very few contraindications to donation.

Local Organ Donor Program #:

Psychiatric Emergencies

HX—Hx recent crisis? Emotional trauma, suicidal, changes in behavior, drug/alcohol abuse? Toxins, head injury, diabetes, sz disorder, sepsis or other illness? Ask about suicidal feelings, intent; does pt. have a plan? Make judgement about whether patient will act on plan. Vitals, with pupil signs, Mental status, oriented? Any odor on breath? Medic alert tags? Any signs of trauma?

✛—**Make sure scene is safe—protect yourself!** Contact OLMC or psychiatric hospital. ABCs, Restrain pt. as needed. If pt. is suicidal do not leave alone. Remove dangerous objects (weapons, pills, etc). Transport in calm, quiet manner, if possible. Consider: O_2, IV, check blood sugar. If low, consider glucose, PO or IV.

Caution—Always suspect hypoglycemia, and look for other medical causes: ETOH, drugs, sepsis, CVA, etc.

Scene Safety

✓ **As you approach, scan the area for hazards such as: hostile persons, dogs, uncontrolled traffic, spilled chemicals, gas, oil, down power lines.**

✓ **Keep your exit routes open.**

✓ **Any weapons present at the scene should be secured.**

✓ **Wear protective gear. Call for more resources if needed.**

Medical Response

CAUTION: **Consider the safety of your crew first!**

1 **Consider staging out of sight until scene is secure**

2 **Make a mental note of physical and weather conditions**

3 **Do not park your vehicle over visible tire tracks**

4 Limit the number of personnel allowed on scene

Crime Scene Access and Treatment

1 **Consult with police regarding best access**

2 **To avoid destroying evidence, select a single route to and from the victim**

3 **When moving the victim, it is important to note:**
   ✓ Location of furniture prior to moving
   ✓ Position of victim prior to moving
   ✓ Status of clothing
   ✓ **Location of any weapons or other articles**
   ✓ Name of personnel who moved items

4 **Consult with police regarding whether to pick up medical debris left over from treatment**

5 **Be conscious of any statements made**

6 **Do Not cut through any holes in patients' clothing**

7 **Place victim on a clean sheet for transport. After transport, obtain the sheet, fold it onto itself, & give to the police**

8 **Write a detailed report regarding your crews actions**

Respiratory Distress

HX—Ask **PAIN QUESTIONS & GENERAL HISTORY**. **Onset of event: was it slow or fast?** Fever? Cough? Is cough productive? Recent respiratory infection? Does patient smoke? (how much?) Record patient's medications. **Assess severity of dyspnea** (mild, moderate, severe); & tidal volume. **Single word sentences? Is cyanosis present?** Level of consciousness? Lung sounds: any wheezing, crackles, rhonchi, diminished sounds? Vitals? Pulse oximetry; **is patient exhausted? Candidate for intubation?** Upper airway obstruction? (stridor, hoarseness, drooling, coughing?) Cx pain? Itching, hives? Numbness of mouth and hands? Signs of CHF: JVD, wet lung sounds (crackles), peripheral edema?

✚—**General treatment—** Position of comfort (usually upright) Give O_2 as needed. **Be prepared to assist ventilations.** Monitor EKG, vitals. Consider IV.

Caution—High flow O_2 can depress respirations in a patient with COPD. Prepare to assist respirations.

✚—**Anaphylaxis:** *See* Allergic Reaction, page 51.

✚—**Asthma:** *Consider nebulized bronchodilator, and / or epinephrine 1:1,000 SQ (0.3 mg – 0.5 mg).*

✚—**COPD:** *Consider nebulized bronchodilator.*

✚—**Pulmonary edema:** *Consider nebulized bronchodilator, furosemide, morphine and sublingual nitroglycerine.*

✚—**Tension Pneumothorax:** Contact OLMC. Lift occlusive dressing, needle thoracentisis. **Rapid transport.**

Lung Sounds

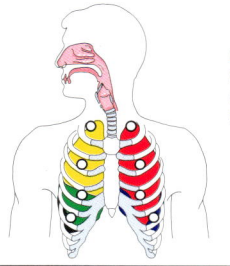

Move stethoscope from apices to bases, comparing sounds from left to right

Disease	Lung Sounds	Other S/Sx; Notes
Asthma	Wheezing; Crackles	Hx allergies, Hx asthma; Pt takes bronchodilators
Bronchitis	Wheezes; Crackles	Recent respiratory tract infection; Smoker
Congestive Heart Failure	Crackles; Wheezes	Pedal edema; Hx CHF; Pt takes Lanoxin, Lasix
Emphysema (COPD)	Wheezing; Rhonchi	Smoker; Pt takes Theophylline, O_2
Foreign Body Obstruction	Stridor; Wheezing	Heard best right over the site of the obstruction
Pneumonia	Scattered crackles; Wheezing	Fever; brown, green, or yellow sputum; Dehydration. Pt takes antibiotics
Pneumothorax	Decreased on one side	Deviated trachea (late); Hyperresonant percussion

NOTE: When in doubt about the cause of the patient's respiratory distress, give oxygen. Hyperventilation of unknown origin can be shock, sepsis, stroke, drug OD.

66

Seizures

❖ **Consider epilepsy, hypoxia, CVA, cardiac origin, ETOH / drug withdrawal, hypoglycemia.**

HX—**onset, length of Sz,** type? previous Hx? Sz meds? Compliance? **Recent head trauma?** What was pt. doing before Sz? Did pt. fall? Bite tongue? Dysrhythmias? Incontinent? Is Sz drug-induced (antidepressant, cocaine)? Medic Alert™? level of consciousness, Head or oral trauma? Focal neurologic signs? H/A? Respiratory status?

✚—**Treatment for Status epilepticus** Keep airway open, consider NPA (do not use EOA/EGTA), O_2, suction, *IV, test blood glucose, consider IV glucose. Transport on side, Monitor EKG, vitals*

Caution—Restrain patient only to prevent injury – protect patient's head. Do not force anything into the mouth. Always check for a pulse after a seizure stops. Most seizures are self-limiting, lasting less than 1–2 minutes.

Shock

HX—Ask **PAIN QUESTIONS & GENERAL HISTORY. Onset?** Associated symptoms: hives, edema, thirst, weakness, dyspnea, cx pain, dizziness when upright, abdominal pain? **Trauma?** Bloody vomitus or stools? Delayed capillary refill? Tachypnea? Syncope? N&V? **Mental status: confusion, restlessness?** Tachycardia, hypotension? **Skin: pale, sweaty, cool.** Signs of pump failure: JVD while upright, crackles, peripheral edema.

✚—Stop hemorrhage if any, Apply direct pressure to wound. Consider pressure point. Place patient supine, O_2 high flow, assist ventilations as needed, start large bore IV, **Don't delay transport to start IV.** (consider intraosseous infusion if unable to start IV). Prevent heat loss. Try to determine the type of shock (hypovolemic, cardiogenic, anaphylactic, septic, neurogenic, etc.). **If trauma, enter patient in Trauma System.** Assess lung sounds. *Monitor EKG,* O_2 sat, vitals, level of consciousness.

Caution—Check lung sounds for crackles a̅ giving IV fluids.

Spinal Injury

HX—MOI, helmet worn? Suspect C-spine injury with head or neck trauma, and with multi-system trauma, or diving/ drowning. Altered mental status? Is there paralysis, weakness, numbness, tingling? Spinal pain with or without movement; point tenderness, deformity, or guarding?

❖Keep airway open. Consider nasopharyngeal airway. Splint neck with C-collar & immobilize the entire spine. Move the patient as a unit and only as necessary. Give O$_2$ *Start large bore IV.* Vitals. **Place patient in Trauma System**.

❖**Caution**— Be prepared to suction and / or move the patient as a unit while immobilized. Consider internal bleeding.

Spinal Innervation

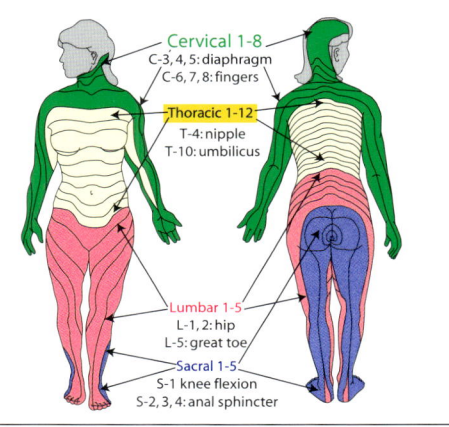

Cervical 1-8
C-3, 4, 5: diaphragm
C-6, 7, 8: fingers

Thoracic 1-12
T-4: nipple
T-10: umbilicus

Lumbar 1-5
L-1, 2: hip
L-5: great toe

Sacral 1-5
S-1 knee flexion
S-2, 3, 4: anal sphincter

Stroke / CVA

HX—Ask **PAIN QUESTIONS & GENERAL HISTORY.** Onset, progression, preceding symptoms (i.e. headache, seizures, confusion, etc.) Past Hx: hypertension? Diabetes? Meds, medic alert tag? **Level of consciousness,** GCS, O₂ sat, chemstrip.

Neurological status: paralysis? Pupils, facial droop, unequal hand grips? Slurred speech, difficulty understanding?

✚—Keep airway open, O₂, assist ventilations if needed. *Start IV. Monitor EKG:* CVA may be 2° to cardiac event, Record Glasgow Coma Score, vitals, Consider hypoglycemia and give glucose only if indicated. **Patient may be a candidate for fibrinolysis. Consider rapid transport**

Caution—Keep airway open, suction & ventilate if needed.

Brain Areas

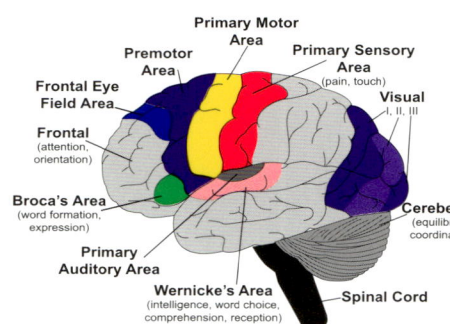

Primary Motor
Area

Premotor
Area

Primary Sensory
Area
(pain, touch)

Frontal Eye
Field Area

Visual
I, II, III

Frontal
(attention,
orientation)

Broca's Area
(word formation,
expression)

Cerebellum
(equilibrium,
coordination)

Primary
Auditory Area

Wernicke's Area
(intelligence, word choice,
comprehension, reception)

Spinal Cord

Fibrinolytic Checklist of Ischemic Stroke

All of the YES boxes and all of the NO boxes must be checked before fibrinolytic therapy can be given.

INCLUSION CRITERIA (all must be YES)

- ❑ Age 18 years or older
- ❑ Clinical Dx: ischemic stroke causing measurable neuro deficit
- ❑ Time of symptom onset will be <3 hrs before fibrinolytic treatment begins

EXCLUSION CRITERIA (all must be NO)

- ❑ Intracranial hemorrhage on noncontrast CT
- ❑ Clinical suspicion subarachnoid bleed, even with normal CT
- ❑ Multilobar infarction on CT > 1/3 cerebral hemisphere
- ❑ Uncontrolled HTN: systolic BP>185 mm Hg or diastolic BP > 110 mm HG of treatment, using repeated measurements, including manual rechecks
- ❑ Hx: intracranial bleed, AV malformation, aneurysm, or neoplasm
- ❑ Witnessed seizure at stroke onset
- ❑ Active internal bleeding or acute trauma (fracture)
- ❑ Known bleeding diathesis, including but not limited to:
- ✓ Platelet count <100,000 / mm^3
- ✓ Patient has received heparin within 48 hours and had an elevated aPTT (greater than upper limit of normal for lab)
- ✓ Current use of anticoagulant (e.g., warfarin sodium) and elevated prothrombin time > 15 seconds, or INR > 1.7
- ✓ Less than three months ago: intracranial or intraspinal surgery, serious head trauma, or previous stroke
- ✓ Recent atterial puncture at a noncompressible site

RELATIVE CONTRADICTIONS (weigh risks vs. benefits)

- ❑ Only minor or rapidly-improving stroke symptoms
- ❑ Within 14 days of major surgery or serious trauma
- ❑ Within 21 days of GI or urinary tract hemorrhage
- ❑ Recent acute MI or Post-MI pericarditis
- ❑ Blood glucose < 50 mg% or > 400 mg%

Posturing

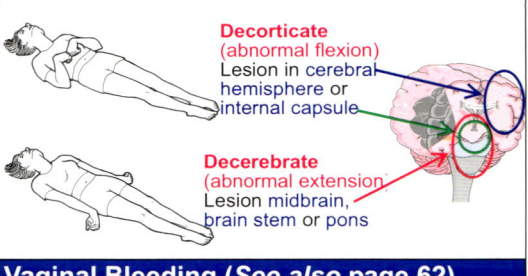

Decorticate
(abnormal flexion)
Lesion in cerebral hemisphere or internal capsule

Decerebrate
(abnormal extension)
Lesion midbrain, brain stem or pons

Vaginal Bleeding (*See also* page 62)

❖**Consider: miscarriage, ectopic pregnancy, CA, trauma.**
HX—Ask **PAIN QUESTIONS & GENERAL HISTORY**.
Cramping? Clots, tissue fragments (bring to ER), **dizziness, weakness**, thirst; (painless bleeding with pregnancy suggests placenta previa). Duration, amount; last menstrual period (normal?); If pt. pregnant: due date? Past Hx: bleeding problems, pregnancies, medications? Vitals and **orthostatic change?** Fever? Evidence of blood loss; **Signs of shock?** vasoconstriction, sweating, altered mental status.
❖**General Treatment:** O₂, *IV large bore, titrated to vitals,* assess vitals, O₂ sat, EKG.
Caution—if miscarriage is suspected, field vaginal exam is generally not indicated.
❖**Postpartum bleeding:** treat for shock, massage uterus to aid contraction, have mother nurse infant, *start large bore IV,* transport without waiting for placenta to deliver. Bring it with you to the hospital. Get vital signs.
❖**Abruptio Placenta:** painful 3rd trimester bleeding; look for hypovolemic shock; give O₂, *start IV,* **Rapid transport.**
❖**Placenta previa:** painless 3rd trimester bleeding; *start IV,* O₂, **Rapid transport.**

Poisons & Overdoses

Please note: this section lists only **some** of the:
- **AKA**—Common brand ®, ™, & "street names"
- **SE**—Common Toxic Side Effects
- **Caution—Primary Cautions**
- **Rx—Prehospital care**
- **Substance Type**

Before administering treatment, consult your Poison Center, the product label or insert, your protocols, and/or your On-Line Medical Resource.

Acids

- **Caustics**

AKA—rust remover; metal polish
SE—pain, GI tract chemical burns, lip burns, vomiting.
Rx—Give milk or water, milk of magnesia, egg white, prevent aspiration. Transport patient in sitting position, if possible.
Caution—Do not induce vomiting. Contact Poison Control Center for more advice.

Acetaminophen

- **Analgesic**

AKA—Tylenol®, APAP
SE—there may be no S/Sx, but acetaminophen is toxic to the liver. N&V, anorexia, RUQ pain, pallor, diaphoresis.
Rx—ABCs, O₂, IV, EKG, fluids for hypotension. Activated charcoal 50 – 100 gm orally. Acetylcysteine may be given in ED.
Caution—Contact Poison Control Center for advice.

Alkalis

- **Caustics**

AKA—Drano®; drain & oven cleaners; bleach
SE—pain, GI tract chemical burns, lip burns, vomiting.
Rx—Give milk or water, prevent aspiration. Transport pt in sitting position, if poss.
Caution—Do not induce vomiting. Call Poison Control Center.

Amphetamines / Stimulants

- **Stimulant**

AKA—methamphetamine, "speed", "crank"
SE—anxiety, ↑HR, arrhythmias, diaphoresis, Sz, N&V, H/A, CVA, HTN, hyperthermia, dilated pupils, psychosis, suicidal.
Rx—*ABCs, O₂, EKG, IV fluids for hypotension. Activated charcoal 50–100 gm orally. Maintain normal body temp. Benzodiazepine as adjunct.*
Caution—Protect yourself against the violent patient.

Antidepressants

- **Mood elevators**

AKA—Norpramin®, Sinequan®, amitriptyline
SE—hypotension, PVCs, cardiac arrhythmias, QRS complex widening, seizures, coma, death.
Rx—*ABCs, O₂, IV, EKG, IV fluids, 1 mEq/kg NaHCO₃ IV, Intubate and hyperventilate.*
Caution—Onset of coma and seizures can be sudden. Do not give ipecac.

Aspirin

- **Analgesic**

AKA—Bayer®, ASA, salicylates
SE—GI bleeding, N&V, LUQ pain, pallor, diaphoresis, shock, tinnitus, ↑RR.
Rx—*ABCs, O₂, IV, EKG, fluids for hypotension. Activated charcoal 50–100 gm orally*
Caution—Conact Poison Control Center for advice.

Barbiturates / Sedatives

- **Hypnotic**

AKA—phenobarbital, "barbs", "downers".
SE—weakness, drowsiness, respiratory depression, apnea, coma, hypotension, bradycardia, hypothermia, APE, death.
Rx—*ABCs, O₂, ventilate, IV fluids for hypotension.*
Caution—Protect the patient's airway.

Carbon Monoxide

- **Odorless Toxic Gas**

Causes—any source of incomplete combustion, such as: car exhaust, fire suppression, and stoves.

SE—H/A, dizziness, DOE, fatigue, tachycardia, visual disturbances, hallucinations, cherry red skin color, ↓ respirations, N&V, cyanosis, altered mental status, coma, blindness, hearing loss, convulsions.

Rx—Remove pt. from toxic environment, ABCs, O₂, transport. Hyperbaric treatment in severe cases.

Caution—Protect yourself from exposure!

Cocaine

- **Stimulant / anesthetic**

AKA—"coke", "snow", "flake", "crack"

SE—H/A, N&V, ↓ RR, agitation, ↑HR, arrhythmias, cx pain, vasoconstriction, AMI, HTN, Sz, vertigo, euphoria, paranoia, vomiting, hyperthermia, tremors, paralysis, coma, dilated pupils, bradycardia, death. APE with IV use.

Rx—ABCs, O2, IV, ET intubation. Consider: benzodiazepine for Sz, lidocaine for PVCs, calcium blocker or beta blocker (labetalol) and nitrates for AMI. Control HTN. Monitor VS and core temp: cool patient if hyperthermic. Minimize sensory stimulation.

Caution—Protect yourself from the violent patient. A "speedball" is cocaine + heroin.

Ecstasy/MDMA (methylenedioxymethamphetamine)

- **Stimulant/Hallucinogen**

AKA—"XTC", "X", "love drug", "MDMA", "Empathy"

SE—euphoria, hallucinations, agitation, teeth grinding (use of pacifiers), nausea, hyperthermia, sweating, HTN, tachycardia, renal and heart failure, dilated pupils, seizures, rhabdomyolysis, DIC, APE, CVA, coma, electrolyte imbalance.

Rx—ABCs, O₂, vitals, *EKG, IV,* cool pt if hyperthermic, intubate if unconscious; benzodiazepine for Sz.

Caution—Do not give beta blockers.

GHB (gamma hydroxy buterate)

- **Depressant**

AKA—"G", "easy lay", "liquid X", "Blue Nitro"

SE—euphoria, sedation, dizziness, myoclonic jerking, N&V, H/A, coma, bradycardia, apnea.

Rx—ABCs, manage airway, ventilate

Caution—A common "date rape" drug.

Hallucinogens

- **Alter perception**

AKA—LSD, psilocybin mushrooms

SE—anxiety, hallucinations, panic, disorientation, N&V.

Rx—Calm and reassure the patient. Be supportive.

Caution—Watch for violent & unexpected behavior.

Hydrocarbons

- **Fuels, oils**

AKA—gasoline, oil, petroleum products

SE—breath odor, SOB, Sz, APE, coma, bronchospasm.

Rx—ABCs, O_2, gastric lavage.

Caution—Do not induce vomiting.

Ketamine (KETALAR®)

- **Dissociative Anesthetic**

AKA—"Special K", "Vitamin K", "horse tranquilizer"

SE—nystagmus, hallucinations, sedation, babbling, tachycardia, respiratory depression, N&V, ego-centrism, paranoia, increased salivation, coma, Sz.

Rx—ABCs, protect airway, monitor VS.

Mushrooms (Amanita)

- **Deadly mushroom**

AKA—Death Angel

SE—N&V, Sz, death.

Rx—ABCs, O_2, IV, benzodiazepine for seizures.

Caution—Protect the patient's airway.

Opiates

- **Narcotic analgesic**

AKA—Dilaudid®, heroin, morphine, codeine, fentanyl
SE—↓ respirations, apnea, ↓ BP, coma, bradycardia, pinpoint pupils, vomiting, diaphoresis.
Rx—ABCs, O₂, ventilate, *intubate, IV fluids for hypotension, naloxone 2 mg IV, IM, SQ, ET, IL.*
Caution—Consider other concurrent overdoses.

Organophosphates

- **Insecticides**

AKA—Malathion®, Diazinon®
SE—SLUDGE (Salivation, lacrimation, urination, defecation, G-I, Emesis), pinpoint pupils, weakness. Bradycardia, sweating, N&V, diarrhea, dyspnea.
Rx—Extricate patient, ABCs, O₂, *Atropine 1–2 mg IV every 5 minutes for bradycardia, hypotension.*
Caution—Protect yourself first! Do not become contaminated.

PCP – Phencyclidine

- **Tranquilizer**

AKA—"Peace Pill", "angel dust", "horse tranquilizer"
SE—nystagmus, disorientation, HTN, hallucinations, catatonia, sedation, paralysis, stupor, mania, tachycardia, dilated pupils, status epilepticus.
Rx—ABCs, O₂, vitals, *IV, EKG.*
Caution—Protect yourself against the violent patient. Examine patient for trauma which may have occurred due to anesthetic effect of PCP.

Rohypnol (flunitrazepam)

- **Benzodiazepine**

AKA—"roofies", "Mexican Valium", "Row-shay"
SE— anterograde amnesia, hypotension, sedation, dizziness, confusion, coma.
Rx—ABCs, manage airway, ventilate, monitor vitals; *Flumazenil IV.*
Caution—One of several "date rape" drugs.

Tranquilizers (Major)

• Antipsychotic

AKA—Haldol®, Navane®, Thorazine®, Compazine®
SE—EPS, dystonias, painful muscle spasms, resp. depression, hypotension, torsades de pointes.
Rx—*50–100 mg diphenhydramine for EPS. ABCs, O2, vitals, EKG. Consider activated charcoal 50–100 gm orally. IV fluids for hypotension. Consider intubation for the unconscious patient.*
Caution—Protect the patient's airway.

Tranquilizers (Minor)

• Anxiolytics

AKA—Valium®, Xanax®, diazepam, midazolam
SE—sedation, weakness, dizziness, tachycardia, hypotension, hypothermia, (↓ respirations with IV use)
Rx—ABCs, monitor vitals; *Flumazenil IV.*
Caution—Coma usually means some other substance or cause is also involved. OD is almost always in combination with other drugs. Protect the patient's airway.

Notes

Emergency Medications

Please note: this section lists only some of the:
- ❖ Primary Indications **Rx–**
- ❖ Primary Contraindications (Contra:),
- ❖ **Dosages (bold),**
- ❖ Common Side Effects (SE:)
- ❖ **Drug Type** for these medications.

Pediatric doses (Peds) are in italics or on page 118.

For complete information, please consult the drug product insert, or an appropriate medical resource.

Abciximab (ReoPro®)—*See page 90*

Activated charcoal

- **Adsorbent**

Rx—Poisoning/overdose: 1 gm/kg PO or by NG tube. (Mix with water to make a slurry)

Contra—do not give before or together with ipecac.
Contact Poison Center for more advice.

SE—constipation.

Adenosine (ADENOCARD®)

- **Antiarrhythmic**

Rx—PSVT: 6 mg (2 ml) **IV rapidly over 1–3 secs.**
[flush with 20cc NS bolus; elevate IV arm]
If no effect in 1–2 min, **give 12 mg** over 1–3 sec.
May repeat 12 mg bolus one more time.

Contra—2° or 3° AV block, VT, sick sinus syndrome.

SE—transient dysrhythmias, facial flushing, dyspnea, chest pressure, hypotension, headache, nausea, bronchospasm.

NOTE: **adenosine is blocked by theophyllines; but potentiated by dipyridamole, carbamazepine.**

Peds: 0.1–0.2 mg/kg IV rapidly, IO up to 6 mg. May double dose if no effect. Max: 12 mg/dose.

Albuterol 0.5% (VENTOLIN®)

•Bronchodilator
Rx—Bronchospasm 2° COPD, Asthma: **1.25–2.5 mg** (0.25–0.5 ml); **mixed in 3 ml saline in nebulizer.**
Contra—tachydysrhythmias.
SE—tachydysrhythmias, anxiety, nausea & vomiting.
Peds: 0.03 ml/kg nebulized; max: 1 ml.

Alteplase (ACTIVASE®, tPA)

• Fibrinolytic
Acute MI (< 12 hours old): 100 mg IV over 3 hrs.
Mix in 100 ml sterile water for 1 mg/ml.

Accelerated 1.5 hour infusion:

• Administer **15 mg IV bolus** (15 ml) over 2 minutes,
• Then give **0.75 mg/kg** (Max: 50 mg) **over next 30 min,**
• Followed by **0.5 mg/kg** (Max: 35 mg) **over next hr.**

Or 3-hour infusion:

• Administer **10 mg IV bolus** (10 ml) **over 2 minutes,**
• Then give **50 mg** (50 ml) **over first hour,**
• Followed by **20 mg/hr** (20 ml/hr) **the next 2 hours.**
Rx—Acute Ischemic Stroke (< 3 hours old): **0.9 mg/kg IV** (Max: 90 mg) **over 1 hour.**
• Give 10% of the dose as an IV bolus over 1 minute,
• Then give the remaining 90% over the next hour.
Rx—Acute Pulmonary Embolism: **100mg IV over 2 hrs.**
Contra—Any within 3 months: • stroke, • AV malformation, • neoplasm, • recent trauma, • aneurysm, • recent surgery. Active internal bleeding w/in 21 days; major surgery or trauma w/in 14 days, aortic dissection, severe HTN, known bleeding disorders, prolonged CPR with thoracic trauma, LP w/in 7 days, arterial puncture at a non-compressible site. *See page 26 for more contraindications.*
SE—reperfusion dysrhythmias, bleeding, shock.

Amiodarone (CORDARONE®)

- **Antiarrhythmic**

Rx—Cardiac Arrest VF / VT: 300 mg IVP. May repeat 150 mg IVP q 3–5 minutes. Max: 2,200 mg/24 hours.

Rx—Stable Wide Complex Tachycardia:

Rapid infusion:

150 mg IV over 10 minutes. May repeat 150 mg IVP q̄ 10 minutes. Max 2,200 mg/24 hrs.

(mix 150 mg in 100 ml; run at 10 ml/min or 600 microdrop/min)

Slow infusion:

360 mg IV over 6 hours.

(mix 1000 mg in 500 ml; run at 30 ml/hr or 30 microdrop/min)

Maintenance infusion:

540 mg IV over 18 hours.

(mix 1000 mg in 500 ml; run at 15 ml/hr or 15 microdrop/min)

Contra—cardiogenic shock, bradycardia, 2°, 3° block; do not use with drugs that prolong QT interval.

SE—vasodilation, ↓BP, ↓HR, AV block, hepatotoxicity, ↑QTc, VF, VT. 40 day half-life.

Peds dose: 5 mg/kg IV/IO.

Amyl nitrite

- **Cyanide Antidote**

Rx—Cyanide poisoning: Administer vapors from crushed inhalant for 30 sec, then administer oxygen for 30 seconds, repeat continuously.

SE—hypotension, H/A, nausea, methemoglobinemia.

Anistreplase (EMINASE®, APSAC)

- Fibrinolytic

Rx—Acute MI (< 12 hrs old): 30 IU IV over 2–5 minutes (mix in 50 ml SW).

Contra—active internal bleeding within 21 days; Any within 3 months: • stroke, • AV malformation, • neoplasm, • aneurysm, • recent trauma, • recent surgery. Major surgery or trauma within 14 days, aortic dissection, severe uncontrolled HTN, known bleeding disorders, prolonged CPR with thoracic trauma, lumbar puncture within 7 days, arterial puncture at a non-compressible site. *See page 26 for additional contraindications.*

SE—reperfusion dysrhythmias, bleeding, shock, H/A, hypotension, allergic reaction, chest pain, N&V.

Aspirin (ASA)

- **Antiplatelet**

Rx—Acute Myocardial Infarction: 160–325 mg P.O. (2–4 chewable children's aspirin tablets).

Contra—allergy. Use caution with: asthma, ulcers, GI bleeding, other bleeding disorders.

SE—GI bleeding.

Atenolol (TENORMIN®)

- **Beta Blocker**

Rx—VT, VF, Atrial fib, Atrial flutter, PSVT, HTN
Rx—Myocardial Salvage for:

- **Acute Anterior MI c̄ HTN & Tachycardia**
- **Large MI < 6 hours old**
- **Refractory Cx Pain or Tachycardia 2° excess sympathetic tone:**

5 mg IV slowly over 5 minutes. Wait 10 minutes, then give another 5 mg IV slowly over 5 minutes.

Contra—CHF, APE, bronchospasm, Hx asthma, ↓HR, 2° or 3° heart block, cardiogenic shock ↓BP.

SE—↓BP, CHF, bronchospasm, ↓HR, cx pain, H/A, N&V.
Calcium blockers may exacerbate side effects.

Atropine sulfate

- **Vagolytic**

Rx—Asystole, PEA: **1 mg IVP**, (2–3 mg ET); q̄ 3–5 minutes; up to 0.04 mg/kg total dose.

Rx—Symptomatic Bradycardia: **0.5–1 mg IVP** q̄ 3–5 minutes; up to 0.04 mg/kg total dose.

Rx—Organophosphate or Carbamate insecticide poisoning: **2–5 mg IV** q̄ 15–30 minutes *(0.05 mg/kg in children) until vital signs improve.*

Rx—Asthma: **0.4–2 mg nebulized in 3 ml saline.**

Rx—RSI (pediatric): **0.02mg/kg. Minimum 0.1mg**

Contra—tachycardia, glaucoma.

SE—dilated pupils, ↑HR, VT, VF, H/A, dry mouth.

Calcium chloride 10%

- **Electrolyte**

Rx—Calcium blocker toxicity; Hypocalcemia with tetany; Hyperkalemia; Hypermagnesemia: **500–1000 mg IV over 5–10 minutes.**

Contra—VF, digitalis toxicity, hypercalcemia.

SE—↓HR, asystole, ↓BP, VF, coronary & cerebral artery spasm, N&V; extravasation causes necrosis.

NOTE: Precipitates with NaHCO3 in IV bag/tubing.

Peds: 10–20 mg/kg (0.1–0.2 mL/kg) IV, IO slowly.

Calcium gluconate 10%

- **Electrolyte**

Rx—Calcium blocker OD; Hypocalcemia; Hyperkalemia; Hypermagnesemia: **500–1000 mg IV slowly.**

Contra—VF, digitalis toxicity, hypercalcemia.

SE—↓HR, ↓BP, VF, arterial spasm; infiltration causes necrosis.

NOTE: Precipitates with NaHCO$_3$ in IV bag/tubing.

Peds: 60–100 mg/kg (0.6–1 mL/kg) IV, IO slowly.

Dalteparin (FRAGMIN®), Enoxaparin (LOVENOX®)—See page 92

Dexamethasone (DECADRON®)

- **Anti-inflammatory**
Rx—Cerebral Edema, Anaphylaxis, COPD, Spinal Trauma: 10–100 mg IV.
Contra—uncontrolled infections, TB, ulcers.
Peds: 0.25–1 mg/kg IV, IO, IM.

Dextrose 50%

- **Nutrient**
Rx—Coma, Hypoglycemia: 25 gm (50 ml) **IV.**
SE—tissue necrosis if extravasation occurs.
Contra—intracerebral bleeding, hemorrhagic CVA.

Diazepam (VALIUM®)

- **Anticonvulsant/sedative**
Rx—Status Epilepticus: 5–10 mg IV slowly.
Rx—Sedation: 5–15 mg IV slowly.
(Rectal diazepam: 0.5 mg/kg via 2" rectal catheter. Flush with 2–3 ml of air after administration.)
Contra—head injury, ↓BP, acute narrow angle glaucoma.
SE—↓ respirations, ↓BP, drowsiness, venous irritation.
NOTE: overdose may be reversed with flumazenil.

Diphenhydramine (BENADRYL®)

- **Antihistamine**
Rx—Allergic Reaction, EPS: 25–50 mg IV, or deep IM.
Contra—asthma, pregnant or lactating females.
SE—sedation, blurred vision, anticholinergic effects.
Peds: 1–2 mg/kg IV, IO slowly, or IM.

Diltiazem (CARDIZEM®)

- **Antiarrhythmic**

Rx—PSVT; Rapid Atrial Fibrillation, Atrial Flutter: 0.25 mg / kg slowly IV over 2 minutes; if no effect in 15 minutes: 0.35 mg/kg IV slowly over 2 minutes.
Drip: 10–15 mg / hr (5 mg/hr for some patients).

Diltiazem (5mg/cc)	Patient Weight in kg					
Bolus Doses in ccs	**50**	**60**	**70**	**80**	**90**	**100**
1st dose: 0.25 mg/kg	2.5cc	3cc	3.5cc	4cc	4.5cc	5cc
2nd dose: 0.35 mg/kg	3.5cc	4.2cc	4.9cc	5.6cc	6.3cc	7cc

[for drip: mix 125 mg (25 cc) in 100 ml IV solution (1 mg/ml) & run at:]

Diltiazem Drip	*mg/hour →*	5 mg	10 mg	15 mg
	microdrops/min →	5 gtt	10 gtt	15 gtt

Contra—2° or 3° block, ↓BP, sick sinus syndrome, VT; WPW or short PR syndrome with atrial fib or atrial flutter. Do not give with oral beta blockers. Do not give with furosemide in same IV line (flush line first).
SE—hypotension, bradycardia, H/A, N&V, CHF, dizziness, weakness. Diltiazem ↑serum digoxin levels.

Droperidol (INAPSINE®)

- **Tranquilizer**

Rx—Chemical Restraint: 0.625–10 mg IV slowly or IM;
Maintenance: 1.25–2.5 mg IV.
Contra—renal or hepatic disease, prolonged QTI.
SE—↓BP, tachycardia, apnea, EPS; VT (torsades).
Peds: 2–12 years: 0.1–0.15 mg/kg IV, IO, IM.

Dobutamine (DOBUTREX®)

- **Inotrope**
Rx—CHF: 2–20 mcg/kg/min.
Mix 250 mg in 250 ml D5W (1 mg/ml) and run at:

mcg/kg/min.	Patient weight in kg											
	2.5	5	10	20	30	40	50	60	70	80	90	100
2 mcg	*	*	1	2	4	5	6	7	8	10	11	12
5 mcg	*	1.5	3	6	9	12	15	18	21	24	27	30
10 mcg	1.5	3	6	12	18	24	30	36	42	48	54	60
15 mcg	2	5	9	18	27	36	45	54	63	72	81	90
20 mcg	3	6	12	24	36	48	60	72	84	96	108	120

microdrops/minute, or ml/hr

Contra—tachydysrhythmias, IHSS, hypovolemia, poison-induced shock, shock with BP < 100.
SE—tachydysrhythmias, VT, VF, HTN, N&V, H/A, AMI.
*Peds: For pediatric infusion, **see** page 118.*

Dopamine (INTROPIN®)

- **Inotrope**
Rx—Hypotension; Bradycardia: 2–20 mcg/kg/min.
Renal Dose: 2–5 mcg/kg/min.
Inotropic Dose: 5–10 mcg/kg/min.
Pressor Dose: >10 mcg/kg/min.
Mix 400 mg in 250 ml D5W (1600mcg/ml) & run at:

mcg/kg/Min.	Patient weight in kg											
	2.5	5	10	20	30	40	50	60	70	80	90	100
2 mcg	*	*	*	1.5	2	3	4	5	5	6	7	8
5 mcg	*	1	2	4	6	8	9	11	13	15	17	19
10 mcg	1	2	4	8	11	15	19	23	26	30	34	38
15 mcg	1.4	3	6	11	17	23	28	34	39	45	51	56
20 mcg	2	4	8	15	23	30	38	45	53	60	68	75

microdrops/minute, or ml/hr

Contra—↑HR, HTN. ↓dose to 1/10th for pts on MAOIs.
SE—tachydysrhythmias, VT, VF, HTN, N & V, H/A, ischemia, AMI.

Extravasation causes tissue necrosis.

Enalaprilat (VASOTEC®)

- ACE Inhibitor / Antihypertensive

Rx—HTN, Acute MI, CHF: 0.625–1.25 mg IV slowly.
(Use lower dose if patient is on diuretics)
Repeat in 1 hr if no response, then 1.25 mg IV $\overline{q}$ 6 hrs.
Contra—renal impairment, pregnancy, lactation.
SE—H/A, dizziness, fatigue, ↓LOC, dyspnea, ↓BP.

Enoxaparin (LOVENOX®)—*See page 91*

Epinephrine (ADRENALIN®)

- **Sympathomimetic**

Rx—Allergic Reaction: 0.3–0.5 mg (0.3–0.5 ml 1:1000) **SQ.**
Peds: 0.01 mg/kg (0.01 ml/kg) SQ—max 0.5 mg
Rx—Anaphylaxis: 0.3–0.5 mg (3–5 ml 1:10,000) **IV.**
Rx—Asthma: 0.3–0.5 mg (0.3–0.5 ml 1:1000) **SQ.**
Rx—Bradycardia / Hypotension: 2–10 mcg/min IV.
(mix 1 mg in 250 ml D5W):

Epinephrine Drip

mcg / min→	2	3	4	5	6	7	8	9	10
microdrops→	30	45	60	75	90	105	120	135	150

Rx—Cardiac arrest: 1 mg IV $\overline{q}$ 3–5 minutes.
Alternative doses for cardiac arrest:
High Dose: 0.2 mg/kg IVP $\overline{q}$ 3 – 5 minutes.
Endotracheal Dose: 2–2.5 mg $\overline{q}$ 3 – 5 minutes.
Continuous Infusion: mix 30 mg in 250 ml NS, or D5W and run at 100 ml/hr (100 microdrops/minute).
Contra—tachydysrhythmias, coronary artery disease
SE—tachydysrhythmias, VT, VF, angina, HTN.

Eptifibatide (INTEGRILIN®)—*See page 90*

Etomidate (AMIDATE®)

- **Sedative/Hypnotic**

Rx—Sedation for RSI: 0.3 mg/kg IV slowly.
Contra—pt < 10 y.o., pregnancy, do not use with ketamine, immunosuppression, sepsis, transplant pt.
SE—apnea, bradycardia, ↓BP, arrhythmias, N&V.

Esmolol (BREVIBLOC®)

- **Antiarrhythmic**

Rx—SVT, Atrial Fib / Flutter: 250*–500* mcg/kg x 1 min. Start drip: 25–50 mcg/kg/min x 4 mins. May ↑ by 25–50 mcg/kg/min; Max: 300 mcg/kg/min. [mix 2.5gm in 250ml D5W]

mcg/kg/ min.	Patient weight in kg								
	40	50	60	70	80	90	100	110	120
*250 mcg	60	75	90	105	120	135	150	165	180
*500 mcg	120	150	180	210	240	270	300	330	360
25 mcg	6	7.5	9	10.5	12	13.5	15	16.5	18
50 mcg	12	15	18	21	24	27	30	33	36
100 mcg	24	30	36	42	48	54	60	66	72
150 mcg	36	45	54	63	72	81	90	99	108
200 mcg	48	60	72	84	96	108	120	132	144
300 mcg	72	90	108	126	144	162	180	198	216

microdrops/minute, or ml/hr

Contra—↓HR, 2°, 3° block, shock, CHF, COPD, asthma.
SE—↓BP, ↓HR, dizziness, cx pain, H/A, bronchospasm.
Calcium blockers exacerbate side effects.

Fentanyl (SUBLIMAZE®)

- **Narcotic analgesic**

Rx—Analgesia: 50–100 mcg IM. Or 2–20 mcg IV slowly over 2 minutes.
Contra—MAOI use, asthma, myasthenia gravis.
SE—↓LOC, ↓BP N &V, bradycardia, apnea.
Peds: 2–10 mcg/kg IV, IO slowly, or IM.

Flumazenil (ROMAZICON®)

- **Antidote**

Rx—Benzodiazepine Overdose: **0.2–0.5 mg IV.**
Maximum dose: 3 mg in a one hour period.
Contra—cyclic antidepressant overdose, status epilepticus, ↑ICP, allergy to benzodiazepines.
SE—Sz, N&V, agitation, withdrawal. Watch for resedation.
Peds: 0.01 mg/kg IV, IO up to 0.2 mg single dose. Maximum total dose: 1 mg.

Fosphenytoin (CEREBYX®)

- **Anticonvulsant**

Rx—Status Epilepticus: **15–20 mg PE /kg IV** (phenytoin equivalents). **Infuse at 100–150 mg PE/ min. Maintenance dose:** 100 mg PE/kg q̄ 8 hrs.
Contra—severe bradycardia, heart block, hypotension, porphyria, renal or hepatic disease.
SE—tinnitus, dizziness, somnolence, H/A, paresthesia, pruritus.
Peds: 20 mg/kg IV, IO, IM.

Furosemide (LASIX®)

- **Diuretic**

Rx—CHF with Pulmonary Edema, Hypertensive Crisis: **0.5–1 mg/kg IV slowly.** Max: 2 mg/kg.
Contra—dehydration, hypokalemia, hepatic coma.
SE—hypokalemia, hypotension, dehydration.
Peds: 1 mg/kg IV, IO slowly.

Glucagon

- ↑ **Blood glucose**

Rx—Hypoglycemia: 0.5–1 mg (or Unit) IM, SQ, IV.
Give carbohydrate such as prompt meal, orange juice, D50%, etc., as soon as the patient is alert and can eat.
Rx—Beta-Blocker OD: 3–10 mg IV (50–150 mcg/kg), followed by drip: 1–5 mg/hour.
Peds: 0.1 mg/kg IV, IO, IM, SQ up to 1 mg.

Glycoprotein IIb/IIIa Inhibitors:

- Antiplatelet

Contra—Active bleeding; surgery or trauma <6 wks, bleeding diathesis. Hx: intracranial bleeding, CA, AV malformation, aneurysm, CVA <30 d. Aortic dissection, pericarditis, severe HTN, use of other GP IIb/IIIa inhibitor. Platelets <150,000.

SE—bleeding, allergy, arrhythmias, thrombocytopenia.

Abciximab (ReoPro®)

Binds c platelets x 48hrs.
Rx—ACS, Unstable Angina, PCI: 0.25 mg/kg IV.
Then 0.125 mcg/kg/min drip (max 10 mcg/minute). Use c heparin.
[for drip: mix 9 mg (4.5cc) in 250 ml IV solution (36 mcg/ml) & run at:]

Patient weight in kg →	50	60	70	80	90	100
Drip: 0.125 mcg/kg/min →	10.4	12.5	14.6	16.7	17	17

microdrops/minute, or ml/hr

Eptifibatide (Integrilin®)

Platelets recover in 4–8 hrs.

Rx—Acute Coronary Syndrome or PCI: 180 mcg/kg IV bolus, followed by 2 mcg/kg/min IV drip*:

[for drip: use premixed vial; 75 mg/100 ml (0.75 mg/ml)]

Patient weight in kg →	50	60	70	80	90	100
Drip: 2 mcg/kg/min →	8 gtt	9.6 gtt	11 gtt	13 gtt	14.4 gtt	16 gtt

microdrops/minute, or ml/hr

*(use 1 mcg/kg/min IV drip if creatinine is 2–4 mg dL)

[for drip: use premixed vial; 75 mg/100 ml (0.75 mg/ml)]

Patient weight in kg →	50	60	70	80	90	100
Drip: 1 mcg/kg/min →	4 gtt	4.8 gtt	5.5 gtt	6.5 gtt	7.2 gtt	8 gtt

microdrops/minute, or ml/hr

Tirofiban (Aggrastat®)

Platelets recover in 4–8 hrs.

Rx—ACS: 0.4 mcg/kg/min IV x 30 mins; then 0.1 mcg/kg/ min x 12–24 hrs p̄ PCI. 1/2 dose if renal insufficiency (CrCl<30)

[mix 25 mg in 500 ml D5W or NS (50 mcg/ml) & run at:]

Patient weight in kg→	50	60	70	80	90	100
Loading: 0.4 mcg/kg/min	24 gtt	29 gtt	34 gtt	38 gtt	43 gtt	48 gtt
Drip: 0.1 mcg/kg/min	6 gtt	7 gtt	8 gtt	10 gtt	11 gtt	12 gtt

microdrops/minute, or ml/hr

Heparin—Unfractionated

• **Anticoagulant**

Rx—Acute MI, Venous Thrombosis: 60 IU/kg IV; max: 4,000 IU bolus; **followed by 12 IU/kg/hr IV drip**; max: 1,000 IU/hr. (Keep PTT 1.5–2 X normal— ~ 50–70 sec).

Heparin Bolus Dose

Patient wt→	50kg	60kg	70kg	80kg	90kg	100kg
Bolus dose	3000U	3600U	4000U	4000U	4000U	4000U

Heparin Drip

Mix 25,000 IU in 500 ml D5W (50 U/ml) & run at:

Patient weight →	50kg	60kg	70kg	80kg	90kg	100kg
IV drip: 12 IU/kg/hr →	12 gtt	14 gtt	17 gtt	19 gtt	20 gtt	20 gtt

microdrops/minute, or ml/hr

Contra—thrombocytopenia, hemorrhagic CVA, aneurysm, severe HTN, bleeding (except DIC), platelets < 100,000/ml.

SE—bleeding, allergy, thrombocytopenia, itching.

Heparin antagonist: protamine sulfate 25 mg IV over 10 minutes (1 mg neutralizes appx. 100 IU heparin). *Peds Bolus: 50 units/kg IV; Drip: 10–20 U/kg/hr.*

Heparin—Low Molecular Weight: Dalteparin (FRAGMIN®), Enoxaparin (LOVENOX®)

Rx—Acute Coronary Syndrome, Non-Q-Wave MI:

Contra—hypersensitivity, allergy to pork products, thrombocytopenia, bleeding.

SE—bleeding, allergy, thrombocytopenia, itching.

Dalteparin (FRAGMIN®)

120 IU /kg Sub-Q b.i.d. x 2–8 days (give with aspirin).

Enoxaparin (LOVENOX®)

1 mg/kg Sub-Q b.i.d. x 2–8 days (give with aspirin).

Ibutilide (CORVERT®)

• **Antiarrhythmic**

Rx—Atrial Fibrillation, Atrial Flutter: 1 mg IV slowly over 10 minutes. For patients < 60kg give 0.01 mg/kg IV slowly over 10 minutes. May repeat in 10 minutes.

Contra—Do not give with class 1a antiarrhythmics such as disopyramide, quinidine, procainamide or class III drugs such as amiodarone, sotalol. Use caution with drugs that prolong the QT interval: phenothiazines, TCAs, and H_1 receptor antagonists.

SE—PVCs, VT, hypotension, heart block, nausea, H/A, tachycardia, QT prolongation, torsades.

Inamrinone (INOCOR®)

• Inotrope/vasodilator
Rx—Acute severe, refractory CHF: 0.75 mg/kg IV slowly over 2–5 min (10–15 minutes in patients with marginal blood pressure). **May repeat p̄ 30 min.**
Maintenance infusion: 2–15 mcg/kg/min.
[mix 3 amps (300 mg) in 240 ml saline = 1 mg/ml.]

mcg/kg/ Minute	Patient weight in kg.									
	20	30	40	50	60	70	80	90	100	110
2 mcg	2.4	3.6	4.8	6	7.2	8.4	9.6	10.8	12	13.2
5 mcg	6	9	12	15	18	21	24	27	30	33
7.5 mcg	9	14	18	23	27	32	36	41	45	50
10 mcg	12	18	24	30	36	42	48	54	60	66
15 mcg	18	28	36	46	54	64	72	82	90	100

microdrops/minute, or ml/hr

Contra—hypotension, IHSS, hypovolemia. **Do not mix with dextrose solutions or furosemide.**
SE—dysrhythmias, ↓BP, N&V, fever, cx pn, myocardial ischemia, hepatotoxicity, thrombocytopenia, burning at infusion site.
*Peds dose: **see** page 118*

Ipratropium .02% (ATROVENT®)

• Bronchodilator
Rx—Bronchospasm, COPD, Asthma: 0.5 mg (2.5 ml) nebulized (with albuterol).
Contra—glaucoma, allergy to soy products or peanuts.
SE—dry mouth, H/A, cough.
Peds: 25 mcg/kg.

IV Fluid Rates in Drops / Minute

IV FLUID RATES IN DROPS / MINUTE					
Drip Set:	**10**	**12**	**15**	**20**	**60***
30 cc/hr	5	6	8	10	30
60 cc/hr	10	12	15	20	60
100 cc/hr	17	20	25	33	100
200 cc/hr	33	40	50	67	200
300 cc/hr	50	60	75	100	300
400 cc/hr	67	80	100	133	400
500 cc/hr	83	100	125	167	500
1000 cc/hr	167	200	250	333	1000

*Standard "microdrip" IV tubing has 60 gtt/cc. (Note that with a microdrip IV set, cc/hr = drops/minute.) A normal "TKO" or "KVO" rate is 30–60 cc/hr.

Ketamine (KETALAR®)

- **Anesthetic/analgesic**

Rx—Anesthesia: 2 mg/kg IV q̄ 10–20 minutes, (or 10 mg/kg IM q̄ 12–25 minutes).

Contra—hypertensive crisis, allergy.

SE—HTN, respiratory depression, ↑HR, hallucinations.

Ketorolac (TORADOL®)

- **NSAID analgesic**

Rx—Analgesia: 15–30 mg IV or 30–60 mg IM.

Contra—allergy to ASA or other NSAIDs. Use caution in kidney or liver disease, COPD, asthma, ulcers, bleeding disorders, coumadin use, elderly, diabetes.

SE—nausea, GI bleeding, edema.

Labetalol (NORMODYNE®)

- **Antihypertensive**

Rx—Severe HTN: 10–20 mg IV over 1–2 minutes.
May repeat or double dose q 10 minutes until a total of 150–300 mg OR start infusion of 2–8 mg/min.

Rx—Drip: Mix 200 mg (40 ml) in 160 ml of D5W for a concentration of 1 mg/ml. Start at 2 mg/minute.

Labetalol Drip (1 mg/ml)

mg/minute →	2 mg	4 mg	6 mg	8 mg
microdrops/minute (ml/hr) →	120 gtt	240 gtt	360 gtt	480 gtt

Contra—asthma, cardiac failure, 2°, 3° block, severe bradycardia, cardiogenic shock, hypotension.
SE—hypotension, nausea, dizziness, sweating.

Lidocaine 2% (XYLOCAINE®)

- **Antiarrhythmic**

Rx—Cardiac Arrest VT/VF: 1–1.5 mg/kg IVP; May repeat c̄ 0.5–0.75 mg/kg IVP q̄ 5–10 mins. Max: 3 mg/kg. Start drip ASAP. **ET dose:** 2–4 mg/kg.

Rx—VT c̄ Pulse: 1–1.5 mg/kg IVP; then 0.5–0.75 mg/kg q̄ 5–10 min. up to 3 mg/kg. Start drip ASAP.

Rx—PVCs: 0.5–1.5 mg/kg IV then 0.5–1.5 mg/kg q̄ 5–10 minutes up to 3 mg/kg. Start drip ASAP.

Rx—Preparalytic (RSI): 1–1.5 mg/kg IV.
Peds: 1.5–2 mg/kg up to 6 y.o.

Drip: 1–4 mg/min. Mix 1 gm in 250 ml D5W & run at:

Lidocaine Drip (4 mg/ml) →

Lidocaine Drip (4 mg/ml) →	1 mg	2 mg	3 mg	4 mg
microdrops/minute (ml/hr) →	15 gtt	30 gtt	45 gtt	60 gtt

IM dose: 300 mg IM (4 mg/kg) of 10% solution.

Contra—2°, 3° block, hypotension, Stokes-Adams Synd. Reduce maintenance infusion by 50% if pt is > 70 y.o., has liver disease, or is in CHF or shock.
SE—Sz, slurred speech, altered mental status.

Lisinopril (PRINIVIL®)

• **ACE Inhibitor / Antihypertensive**
Rx—Hypertension, AMI: 5 mg / day PO. Double dose to 10 mg/day after 48 hours, and give for 6 wks.
Contra—renal impairment, angioedema, pregnancy, hypovolemia.
SE—H/A, dizziness, fatigue, nausea.

Lorazepam (ATIVAN®)

• **Anticonvulsant/sedative**
Rx—Status Epilepticus: 2–4 mg slowly IV*, or IM.
Rx—Anxiety, Sedation: 0.05 mg/kg up to 4 mg IM.
Contra—Acute narrow-angle glaucoma.
SE—Apnea, N & V, drowsiness, restlessness, delirium; be prepared to ventilate patient.

NOTE: overdose may be reversed with flumazenil.

Peds: 0.05–0.2 mg/kg IV*, IO* slowly, or IM.

*For IV or IO use, dilute 1:1 in NS, D5%W, or SW.

Magnesium sulfate 10%

• **Electrolyte**
Rx—Cardiac Arrest (Torsades, Hypomagnesemia): 1–2 gm IVP (5–10 gm may be required).
Rx—Torsades c̄ a Pulse: 1–2 gm IV over 5–60 mins. (mix in 50 ml D5W). Start drip of 0.5–1 gm /hr and titrate.
Rx—Acute MI: 1–2 gm IV over 5–60 mins. (mix in 50 ml D5W). Start drip: 0.5–1 gm/hr; run for up to 24 hrs.
Rx—Seizures 2° Eclampsia: 1–4 gm IV slowly.
Rx—Magnesium Deficiency: 0.5–1 gm / hr.
Contra—renal disease, heart block, hypermagnesemia.
SE—hypotension, asystole, cardiac arrest, respiratory and CNS depression, flushing, sweating.
Peds: 25–50 mg/kg IV, IO over 10–20 min. Max: 2 gm.

Mannitol 20%

• Osmotic diuretic
Rx—Cerebral Edema with ↑ ICP: 1–2 gm/kg IV over 30 minutes. May repeat if no effect.
Contra—renal impairment, severe dehydration, severe heart disease, pulmonary edema.
SE—CHF, acidosis, Sz, cx pain, ↑HR, electrolyte depletion, dehydration, ↓BP, coma, hyperosmolality, H/A.
Peds: 1 gm/kg IV, IO slowly over 30 minutes.

Meperidine (DEMEROL®)

• Analgesic
Rx—Analgesia: 50–100 mg IM, SQ or slowly IV.
Contra—patients receiving MAO inhibitors.
SE—sedation, apnea, hypotension, ↑ICP, N&V, ↑HR.
Peds: 1 mg/kg IV, IO, IM, SQ.

Metaproterenol 5% (ALUPENT®)

• Bronchodilator
Rx—Bronchospasm 2° to COPD, Asthma: 10–15 mg (0.2–0.3 ml) **nebulized in 3 ml saline.**
Contra—↑tachydysrhythmias.
SE— ↑HR, anxiety, N&V.
Peds: < 2 y.o. = 0.1 ml; 2–9 y.o. = 0.2 ml; >9 y.o. = 0.3 ml

Methylprednisolone (Solu-Medrol®)

- **Steroid**
- **Rx—Asthma: 40–250 mg IV.**
- **Rx—Spinal Cord Trauma: 30 mg/kg IV.**
- **Contra—**GI Bleed, diabetes, seizures, systemic fungal infection.
- **SE—**euphoria, peptic ulcer, hyperglycemia, hypokalemia.
- *Peds: Asthma: 2 mg/kg IV, IO, IM.*
- *Peds: Spinal cord injury: 30 mg/kg IV, IO, IM.*

Metoprolol (LOPRESSOR®)

- **Beta Blocker**
- **Rx—VT, VF, Atrial fib, Atrial flutter, PSVT, HTN:**
- **Rx—Myocardial Salvage for:**
  - **Acute Anterior MI c̄ HTN & Tachycardia**
  - **Large MI < 6 hours old**
  - **Refractory Cx Pain or Tachycardia 2° excess sympathetic tone:**
- **5 mg IV slowly over 2–5 minutes, repeated q̄ 5 minutes to a total of 15 mg.** Then 50 mg orally bid for at least 24 hrs, thereafter increased to 100 mg bid.
- **Contra—**CHF, APE, bronchospasm, bradycardia, hypotension, cardiomegaly, thyrotoxicosis, Hx asthma.
- **SE—**↓BP, CHF, bronchospasm, ↓HR, cx pain, H/A, N&V.
- **Calcium blockers may potentiate side effects.**

Midazolam (VERSED®)

- **Sedative**
Rx—Seizures: 2.5 mg IV, May repeat in 5 minutes. (If unable to start IV, may give 5 mg IM).
Rx—Sedation: 0.1 mg/kg IV, max single dose 5 mg.
Contra—acute narrow angle glaucoma, shock.
SE—respiratory depression, ↓BP, ↓HR, H/A, N&V.
May reverse with flumazenil.
Peds: 0.1 mg/kg IV, max: 2.5 mg/dose. May repeat. (if unable to start IV, may give 0.2 mg/kg IM, max: 5 mg).

Morphine Sulfate

- **Analgesic**
Rx—Analgesia; Pulmonary Edema: 2–5 mg IV, IM, SQ. May repeat $\bar{q}$ 5 minutes up to 10 mg.
Contra—head injury, exacerbated COPD, depressed resp. drive, hypotension, acute abdomen, ↓LOC.

NOTE: overdose may be reversed with naloxone.

SE—resp. depression, ↓BP, ↓LOC, N & V, ↓HR.
Peds: 0.1–0.2 mg/kg IV, IO, IM, SQ.

Nalmefene (REVEX™)

- **Opioid Antagonist**
Rx—Narcotic Overdose: 0.5 mg / 70 kg IV, IM, SQ. [Single IM dose: 1 mg.] Can give second IV dose in 2–5 minutes: **1 mg / 70 kg IV.** Maximum total IV dose is 1.5 mg. (Give over 60 sec. in renal failure.)
Contra—Use extreme caution if narcotic dependence is suspected. May try 0.1 mg IV to test for withdrawal symptoms.
SE—acute withdrawal s/s, N&V, tachycardia, HTN.

Naloxone (NARCAN®)

- **Narcotic antagonist**

Rx—Opiate Overdose; Coma: 2 mg IV, IM, SQ, ET.
Repeat if needed up to 10 mg total dose.

Contra—do not use on a newborn if the mother is addicted to narcotics; may cause withdrawal.

SE—withdrawal symptoms in the addicted patient.

Nesiritide (NATRECOR®)

- **Vasodilator**

Rx—CHF: 2 mcg/kg IV, followed by an infusion of 0.01 mcg/kg/min (0.1 mL/kg/hour).
Mix 1.5 mg in 250 ml of D5W, or NS, for a concentration of 6 mcg/ml.

Nesiritide Bolus Dose

Patient weight →	60kg	70kg	80kg	90kg	100kg	110kg
Bolus dose →	20 cc	23 cc	27 cc	30 cc	33 cc	37 cc

Nesiritide Drip

Patient weight →	60kg	70kg	80kg	90kg	100kg	110kg
IV drip: 0.1 mL/kg/hr →	6 gtt	7 gtt	8 gtt	9 gtt	10 gtt	11 gtt

(microdrops/minute, ml/hr)

Contra—hypotension, cardiogenic shock, valvular stenosis, low cardiac filling pressures.

SE—hypotension, azotemia, headache, anxiety, N&V.

Nicardipine (CARDENE®)

- **Calcium blocker**

Rx—HTN: 5–20 mg / 1 hr. Mix 50 mg in 230 ml D5W for 200 mcg/ml. Run at 25–100 ml/hr.

mg/hour →	5 mg	10 mg	15 mg	20 mg
Ml/hour (gtt/hour) →	25 ml	50 ml	75 ml	100 ml

Contra—hypotension, aortic stenosis. Caution with renal failure and hepatic dysfunction. Don't mix with RL.

SE—edema, hypotension, dizziness, H/A, tachycardia, N&V, facial flushing, vein irritation: change IV site $\overline{q}$ 12hrs.

Nitrates:

- **Vasodilators**

Rx—ACS; Angina; Hypertension; CHF with APE:

Contra— ↓BP, hypovolemia, intracranial bleeding, aortic stenosis, right ventricle infarction, severe bradycardia or tachycardia, recent use of Viagra®, Cialis® or Levitra®.

SE—HA, hypotension, syncope, tachycardia, flushing.

Nitroglycerin tablets (NITROSTAT®)

0.3–0.4 mg SL, may repeat in 3–5 minutes, (max: 3 doses).

Nitroglycerin paste (NITRO-BID®)

1–2 cm of paste (6–12 mg) **topically.**

Nitroglycerin spray (NITROLINGUAL®)

1–2 sprays (0.4–0.8 mg) **under the tongue.**

Nitroglycerin IV (TRIDIL®)

10–200 mcg / minute. Increase by 5–10 mcg/min q 5 min. until desired effect. Mix 25 mg in 250 ml D5W (100 mcg/ml) & run at:

Dose in mcg/min		microdrops/minute (or ml/hr)	Dose in mcg/min		microdrops/minute (or ml/hr)
5 mcg	=	3 gtts/min.	110 mcg	=	66 gtts/min.
10 mcg	=	6 gtts/min.	120 mcg	=	72 gtts/min.
20 mcg	=	12 gtts/min.	130 mcg	=	78 gtts/min.
30 mcg	=	18 gtts/min.	140 mcg	=	84 gtts/min.
40 mcg	=	24 gtts/min.	150 mcg	=	90 gtts/min.
50 mcg	=	30 gtts/min.	160 mcg	=	96 gtts/min.
60 mcg	=	36 gtts/min.	170 mcg	=	102 gtts/min.
70 mcg	=	42 gtts/min.	180 mcg	=	108 gtts/min.
80 mcg	=	48 gtts/min.	190 mcg	=	114 gtts/min.
90 mcg	=	54 gtts/min.	200 mcg	=	120 gtts/min.
100 mcg	=	60 gtts/min.			

NOTE: use glass IV bottle and non-PVC IV tubing.

Nitroprusside (NIPRIDE®)

- **Vasodilator**

Rx—Hypertensive Crisis; CHF: 0.1–10 mcg/kg/min. Start at 0.1 mcg/kg/min and titrate q 3–5 minutes until desired effect. Mix 50 mg in 250 ml D5W (200 mcg/ml) & run at:

mcg/ kg/min	Patient weight in kg											
	2.5	5	10	20	30	40	50	60	70	80	90	100
0.1 mcg	*	*	0.3	0.6	0.9	1.2	1.5	1.8	2	2.4	2.8	3
0.5 mcg	*	*	1.5	3	4.5	6	7.5	9	10	12	14	15
1 mcg	*	1.5	3	6	9	12	15	18	21	24	27	30
2 mcg	1.5	3	6	12	18	24	30	36	42	48	54	60
4 mcg	3	6	12	24	36	48	60	72	84	96	108	120
8 mcg	6	12	24	48	72	96	120	144	168	192	216	240
10 mcg	7.5	15	30	60	90	120	150	180	210	240	270	300

microdrops/minute, or ml/hr

Contra—compensatory HTN, hypotension, aortic stenosis, recent use (within 24 hrs) of Viagra™, Cialis™, Levitra™.

SE—hypotension, tachycardia, thiocyanate toxicity, hypoxemia, CO_2 retention, H/A, N&V.

NOTE: Wrap IV set in foil or other opaque cover.

*Peds: for pediatric infusion **see** page 118.*

Nitrous Oxide (NITRONOX®)

- **Analgesic**

Rx—Analgesia / Sedation: give mask to patient and allow to self-administer.

Contra— ↓LOC, cyanosis, acute abdomen, shock, ↓BP, pneumothorax, cx trauma, pts who need > 50% O_2.

SE—drowsiness, euphoria, apnea.

NOTE: Ventilate patient area during use.

Ondansetron (ZOFRAN®)

• **Antinauseant**
Rx—Nausea & Vomiting: 4 mg IV slowly, or IM.
Contra—Hypersensitivity to dolasetron, granisetron.
May precipitate with bicarb.
SE—H/A, diarrhea, FV, dizziness, pain, SZ, EPS.
Peds: 0.1 mg/kg slow IV, or IM. Max: 4 mg.

Oxytocin (PITOCIN®)

• ↑ **Uterine contractions**
Rx—Postpartum Hemorrhage: 10 units IM p̄
placenta delivers. Or mix 10–40 units in 1000 ml
balanced salt solution and titrate to control uterine
bleeding.
Contra—rule out multiple fetuses before administration.
SE—HTN, dysrhythmias.

Pancuronium (PAVULON®)

• **Paralytic**
Rx—Paralysis to facilitate tracheal intubation:
0.04–0.1 mg/kg IVP (onset 3 minutes; recovery:
30–45 minutes). Maintenance: 0.01 mg / kg q̄
60 minutes.
Contra—1st trimester pregnancy; use reduced dose in
newborns, myasthenia gravis.
SE—apnea, prolonged paralysis, tachycardia, PVCs,
hypotension, hypertension, bradycardia.

Phenytoin (DILANTIN®)

- **Anticonvulsant**

Rx—Seizures: 15–18 mg/kg (max 25–50 mg/min).
Contra—hypoglycemic seizures (give glucose), ↓HR, 2° & 3° heart block, CHF, ↓respirations, impaired hepatic or renal function, ↓BP, hyperglycemia.
SE—lethargy, H/A, irritability, restlessness, vertigo, hypotension, bradycardia, anorexia.

Caustic to veins: use central line if possible.

Peds: 15–20 mg/kg over 30 minutes. Max: 1 gm.

Phenobarbital (LUMINAL®)

- **Anticonvulsant**

Rx—Status Epilepticus: 100–250 mg IV slowly, or IM.
Contra—porphyria, pulmonary or hepatic dysfunction.
SE—respiratory depression, hypotension, coma, N&V.
Peds: 10–20 mg/kg IV, IO slowly, or IM. May repeat.

Procainamide (PRONESTYL®)

- **Antiarrhythmic**

Rx—Cardiac Arrest VF/VT: 50 mg / minute IV drip (max dose: 17 mg/kg.)
Rx—A-Fib, VT; PSVT c̄ WPW: 20 mg / minute IV until dysrhythmia is converted, hypotension or QRS/ QT widening develops, or 17 mg/kg has been given.
Drip: 1–4 mg/min. Mix 1 gm in 250 ml D5W & run at:

Procainamide Drip			
mg/minute →	1 mg	2 mg	3 mg	4 mg
microdrops/ minute (ml/hr) →	15 gtt	30 gtt	45 gtt	60 gtt

Contra—2° & 3° AV block, torsades de pointes, lupus, digitalis toxicity, myasthenia gravis.
SE—PR, QRS, & QT widening, AV block, cardiac arrest, hypotension, Sz, N & V.
Peds: 15 mg/kg IV, IO over 30–60 minutes;
Peds drip: 20–80 mcg/kg/minute.

Promethazine (PHENERGAN®)

- **Antiemetic/Sedative**
Rx—N&V: 12.5–25 mg IV / IM, or 25 mg PO.
Rx—Sedation: 25–50 mg IV / IM / PO.
Contra—allergy to antihistamines and phenothiazines, lactating females, MAOI use, COPD, HTN, pregnancy.
SE—Drowsiness, viscous bronchial secretions, urinary urgency.
Peds: N&V: 1 mg/kg PO;
Peds: Sedation: 12.5–50 mg PO, PR.

Propranolol (INDERAL®)

- **Beta Blocker**
Rx—VT, VF, Atrial fib, Atrial flutter, PSVT, HTN:
Rx—Myocardial Salvage for:
- **Acute Anterior MI c̄ HTN & Tachycardia**
- **Large MI < 6 hours old**
- **Refractory Cx Pain or Tachycardia 2° excess sympathetic tone:**
1–3 mg IV slowly over 2–5 minutes. Repeat dose after 2 minutes to a total of 0.1 mg/kg. Then 180–320 mg/day orally in divided doses.
Contra—CHF, APE, bronchospasm, Hx asthma, COPD, bradycardia, 2° or 3° heart block, hypotension, cardiogenic shock.
SE—hypotension, CHF, bronchospasm, bradycardia, dizziness, cx pain, headache, N & V. **Use of calcium blockers may potentiate side effects.**

Oxygen

	LITERS / MIN	O$_2$ Delivered
Nasal Cannula	1	24%
	2	28%
	4	36%
	6	44%
NRB Mask	10	80%
	15	90%
Pocket Mask	Mouth-to-Mask	17%
	10	50%
	15	80%
	30	100%
Bag-Valve-Mask (with reservoir)	Room air	21%
	10	90%
	15	95%
Positive Pressure	100	100%

Contra—COPD pts may become apneic with high flow O$_2$.

Pulse Oximetry

Ranges	Prehospital Treatment
Normal: 95-99%	
Mild hypoxia: 91–94%	Give oxygen
Moderate hypoxia: 86–90%	Give 100% oxygen
Severe hypoxia: ≤ 85%	**100% oxygen, ventilate**

Falsely low SpO$_2$ readings may be caused by:
• Cold extremities • Hypothermia • Hypovolemia
Falsely high SpO$_2$ readings may be caused by:
• Anemia • Carbon monoxide poisoning
If in doubt, give oxygen in spite of a normal SpO$_2$.

O₂ Tank Capacities

Tank	Capacity	@15 Lpm	10 Lpm	6 Lpm	2 Lpm
C	240 L	16 min	24 min	40 min	2 hr
D	360 L	24 min	36 min	1 hr	3 hr
E	625 L	41 min	1:02h	1:44h	5:12h
M	3,000 L	3:20h	5:00h	8:20h	25hr
G	5,300 L	5:53h	8:50h	14:43h	44:10h
H	6,900 L	7:40h	11:30h	19:10h	57:30h

Reteplase (RETAVASE®)

• Fibrinolytic
Rx—Acute MI (< 12 hours old): 10 units IV over 2 min. Repeat dose in 30 min. (Flush with NS $\overline{a}$ & $\overline{p}$).
Contra—active internal bleeding; Any within 3 months: • stroke, • AV malformation, • neoplasm, • aneurysm, • recent trauma, • recent surgery. Bleeding disorders, LP within 7 days. *See page 26 for additional contraindications.*
SE—dysrhythmias, bleeding, ↓BP, shock, Fv, allergy.

Sodium bicarbonate 8.4%

• Alkalinizer
Rx—Cardiac Arrest c̄ Good Ventilation: 1 mEq/kg IV, (1 ml/kg) followed by 0.5 mEq/kg q̄ 10 minutes.
Rx—Hyperkalemia; OD of: Tricyclic, Phenobarbital, Diphenhydramine, ASA, Cocaine: 1 mEq/kg IV.
SE—metabolic alkalosis, ↓K⁺, fluid overload.
Must ventilate patient after administration.

Streptokinase (STREPTASE®)

- Fibrinolytic

Rx—Acute MI (< 12 hours old): 1,500,000 IU infused over 60 minutes.

Rx—Pulmonary Embolism: 250,000–600,000 IU over 30 mins. Follow with infusion of 100,000 IU/hr.

Contra—active internal bleeding within 21 days. Surgery or trauma within 14 days. Aortic dissection, severe HTN, bleeding disorders, prolonged CPR with thoracic trauma, lumbar puncture within 7 days, arterial puncture at a non-compressible site. Any w/in 3 months: • stroke, • AV malformation, • neoplasm, • aneurysm, • recent trauma, • recent surgery. Streptokinase use w/in past 2 yrs.

SE—reperfusion dysrhythmias, bleeding, shock, H/A, hypotension, allergic reaction, chest pain, N&V, Fv.

Succinylcholine (ANECTINE®)

- Paralytic

Rx—Paralysis to facilitate ET intubation: 1–2 mg/kg IV. (onset: 1 minute; recovery: 4–6 minutes)

[IM dose: 3–4 mg/kg, max: 150 mg. (onset: 2–3 min)]

Contra—Acute narrow angle glaucoma, penetrating eye injuries, burns > 8 hrs, massive crush injury.

SE—Apnea, malignant hyperthermia, dysrhythmias, ↓HR, HTN, ↓BP, arrest, ↑K^+, intraocular pressure.

Tenecteplase (TNKase)

- Fibrinolytic

Rx—Acute MI (< 12 hours old): 30–50 mg IV.

for bolus: mix 50 mg vial in 10 ml SW (5 mg/ml) & give:

Patient weight in kg →	50	60	70	80	90	100
Bolus dose in ccs: →	6 cc	7 cc	7 cc	8 cc	9 cc	10 cc	10 cc

Contra—previous hemorrhagic stroke; other CVA within 1 year, intracranial CA, internal bleeding, aortic dissection; *See page 26 for additional contraindications.*

SE—dysrhythmias, bleeding, ↓BP, shock, CHF, APE.

Thiamine (vitamin B1)

• Nutrient
Rx—Co-administration with D50%W in patients suspected of malnutrition or thiamine deficiency (starvation, severe alcoholism): **100mg slow IV or IM.**
Contra—hypersensitivity. SE: N&V, hypotension.
SE—N&V, hypotension

Tirofiban (AGGRASTAT®)—*See* page 90

Vasopressin (PITRESSIN®)

• Vasopressor
Rx—Cardiac Arrest (VF/VT): **40 U IVP / IO**
Contra—chronic nephritis c̄ nitrogen retention, migraine, epilepsy, CHF, asthma, CAD, pregnancy, lactation.
SE—IV site pain, stomach cramps, N&V, angina, diarrhea, trembling, eructation, pallor, confusion, hives, wheezing.

Vecuronium (NORCURON®)

• Paralytic
Rx—Paralysis / ET intubation: **0.1 mg/kg IVP** (onset: 1 min; recovery: 45 mins). **Maintenance:** 0.01–0.05 mg/kg.
Contra—newborns, myasthenia gravis.
SE—apnea, weakness.
Peds: 0.1–mg/kg IV, IO.

Verapamil (ISOPTIN®)

- **Antiarrhythmic**

Rx—PSVT, Rapid Atrial Fibrillation, Atrial Flutter: 2.5–5 mg IV slowly. (5–10 mg q̄ 15 min. Max: 30 mg)

Drip: 1-10 mg/hr. Mix 100 mg in 250 ml D5W (0.4 mg/ml).

mg/hour →	1	2	3	4	5	6	7	8	9	10
microdrops/min →	2.5	5	7.5	10	12.5	15	17.5	20	22.5	25

Contra—WPW or short PR syndrome c̄ A-Fib or A-Flutter, 2° or 3°block, V-Tach, ↓BP, shock, IV beta blocker use, sick sinus syndrome, CHF, children < 12 mos.

SE—hypotension, AV block, bradycardia, asystole.
Peds: 0.1–0.2 mg/kg IV, IO slowly. Max: 10 mg/dose.

Notes

Notes

Pediatric Pulseless Arrest
(confirm cardiac rhythm in more than one lead)

Determine pulselessness and Begin CPR, Give O₂, Attach ECG

VF or pulseless VT	Asystole / PEA

VF or pulseless VT

↓

↗ **Defibrillate 2 J/kg (manual)**
or AED if > 1 y.o.
Continue CPR immediately
(5 cycles of 15:2*)
with 100% oxygen
Secure airway when possible, ventilate
with oxygen; Obtain IV or IO access

↓

Still VF/VT? ↗ **Defibrillate 4 J/kg**
Continue CPR immediately
(5 cycles of 15:2*)

↓

Epinephrine IV/IO: 0.01 mg/kg
(1:10,000, 0.1 mL/kg) q̄ 3–5 minutes
OR
ET: 0.1 mg/kg (1:1,000, 0.1 mL/kg)
Identify and treat causes

↓

Still VF/VT? ↗ **Defibrillate 4 J/kg**
Continue CPR immediately
(5 cycles of 15:2*)

↓

Amiodarone 5 mg/kg IV, IO, *or:*
Lidocaine 1 mg/kg IV, IO or ET, *or:*
Magnesium 25-50 mg/kg IV, IO
(for Torsades, max: 2 gms)

↓

Still VF/VT? ↗ **Defibrillate 4 J/kg**
Continue CPR immediately
(5 cycles of 15:2*)

↓

Verify: ET tube placement, paddle
position / contact

Asystole / PEA

↓

Continue CPR immediately
(5 cycles of 15:2*)
Secure airway when possible,
ventilate with oxygen; Obtain IV
or IO access

↓

Epinephrine IV/IO: 0.01 mg/kg
(1:10,000, 0.1 mL/kg)
q̄ 3–5 minutes
OR
ET: 0.1 mg/kg
(1:1,000, 0.1 mL/kg)

↓

Identify and treat causes:

↓

Verify: ET tube placement;

↓

Identify and treat causes:

Severe hypoxemia?
Severe acidosis?
Severe hypovolemia?
Tension pneumothorax?
Cardiac tamponade?
Profound hypothermia?
Electrolyte imbalance?
Drug overdose?
Embolism?
Severe hypoglycemia?
Trauma?

*After ET intubation, give
8-10 breaths / min during
CPR.

112

Pediatric Bradycardia
(with a pulse, but symptomatic)

Assess & Support ABCs
Secure airway, Administer 100% oxygen
Start IV or IO, Assess vital signs, attach ECG

Severe cardiorespiratory compromise?
(poor perfusion, hypotension, respiratory difficulty)

NO ← → YES

Observe,
Support ABCs,
Consider consult with
expert

Oxygenate, ventilate, intubate!
Do CPR if
HR < 60/min in an infant/ child
in spite of good oxygenation
and ventilation

Epinephrine q̄ 3–5 minutes
IV / IO: 0.01 mg/kg (1:10,000, 0.1 mL/kg)*
ET: 0.1 mg/kg (1:1,000, 0.1 mL/kg)*
Repeat every 3–5 minutes at the same dose

Atropine 0.02 mg/kg IV, IO, ET for increased vagal tone or
primary AV block (minimum dose: 0.1 mg)
(maximum single dose: 0.5 mg for child; 1.0 mg for adolescent)
May be repeated once (max. total dose: child 1 mg;
adolescent 2 mg)

Consider Pacing

If arrest develops *See Pediatric Pulseless Arrest (page 112)*

Identity and treat causes:

Hypoxemia?	Acidosis?	Hypothermia?
Hypovolemia?	Head Injury?	Overdose?
Tension pneumothorax?		Heart block?
Electrolyte imbalance?	Cardiac tamponade?	Trauma?
		Hypoglycemia?

Pediatric bradycardia is usually the result of hypoxia

Pediatric Tachycardia
with Poor Perfusion

Assess ABCs (start CPR if no pulse)
Secure airway, Administer 100% oxygen
Start IV or IO, Assess vital signs, Attach 12-lead ECG,
Evaluate the tachycardia; Identify and treat causes below*

QRS Duration?

Normal for age (≤ 0.08 sec.)   **Wide for age (>0.08 sec)**

Probably Sinus Tach if:
Compatible history?
Normal P waves?
HR varies with activity?
Variable R-R c̄ normal PR?
Infant HR <220/min?
Child HR <180/min?

Otherwise, probably SVT
Consider vagal maneuvers
(but do not delay cardioversion)
↓
Adenosine 0.1 mg/kg IVP/IO
(6 mg max dose)
May repeat with 0.2 mg/kg
(12 mg max dose) *OR:*
↓
⚡ **Synchronized cardioversion**
(0.5–1.0 J/kg; may increase to
2 J/kg if initial dose fails.
Sedate if possible, but do not
delay cardioversion)
↓
Consult expert
Amiodarone 5 mg/kg IV
Over 20–60 minutes, *OR:*
Procainamide 15 mg/kg IV
Over 30–60 minutes

Possible V-Tach
⚡ **Cardioversion STAT**
(0.5–1.0 J/kg;
May increase to
2 J/kg if initial dose fails.
Sedate if possible, but do
not delay cardioversion)
May attempt Adenosine
0.1 mg/kg IVP/IO (6 mg max dose)
but do not delay cardioversion
↓
Consult expert
Amiodarone 5 mg/kg IV
Over 20–60 minutes, *OR:*
Procainamide 15 mg/kg IV
Over 30–60 minutes

*Identify and treat causes:
Hypoxemia?
Hypothermia?
Hypovolemia?
Hypoglycemia?
Acidosis?
Tension pneumothorax?
Cardiac tamponade?
Toxins/Drugs?
Electrolyte imbalance?
Trauma? Embolism?

Pediatric Medications

Age	Preterm	Term	6 mos	1 yr	3 yrs	6 yrs	8 yrs	10 yrs	11 yrs	12 yrs	14 yrs
Weight (pounds)	3 lbs	7.5 lbs	15 lbs	22 lbs	33 lbs	44 lbs	55 lbs	66 lbs	77 lbs	88 lbs	99 lbs
Weight (kilograms)	1.5 kg	3.5 kg	7 kg	10 kg	15 kg	20 kg	25 kg	30 kg	35 kg	40 kg	45 kg
Length (inches)	16"	21"	26"	31"	39"	46"	50"	54"	57"	60"	64"
Length (cm)	41 cm	53 cm	66 cm	79 cm	99 cm	117 cm	127 cm	137 cm	145 cm	152 cm	163 cm
Heart Rate	140	125	120	120	110	100	90	90	85	85	80
Respirations	40-60	40-60	24-36	22-30	20-26	20-24	18-22	18-22	16-22	16-22	14-20
Systolic BP	50-60	60-70	60-120	65-125	100	100	105	110	110	115	115
ET Tube Size (mm)	2.5, 3.0	3.5	3.5	4.0	4.5	5.5	6.0	6.5	6.5	7.0	7.0
LMA Size	1	1	1½	1-1½	2	2-2½	2½	2½-3	3	3	3
Suction catheter size	5-6 Fr	8 Fr	8 Fr	8 Fr	8 Fr	10 Fr	10 Fr	10 Fr	10 Fr	10 Fr	10 Fr
Nasogastric tube size	5 Fr	8 Fr	8 Fr	10 Fr	10 Fr	12 Fr	14 Fr	14 Fr	14 Fr	14 Fr	16 Fr
Defibrillation: 2 J/kg, 4 J/kg	3, 6 J	7, 14 J	14, 28 J	20, 40	30, 60	40, 80	50, 100	60, 120	70, 140	80, 160	90, 180
Synchron Shock: 0.5-1 J/kg	1-2 J	2-4 J	4-7 J	5-10 J	8-15	10-20	13-25	15-30	18-35	20-40	23-45
Fluid challenge (LR, NR, NS) 20 ml/kg IV, IO [Neonates-10 ml/kg]	15 ml	35 ml	140 ml	200 ml	300 ml	400 ml	500 ml	600 ml	700 ml	800 ml	900 ml

Age	Preterm	Term	6 mos	1 yr	3 yrs	6 yrs	8 yrs	10 yrs	11 yrs	12 yrs	14 yrs
Adenosine (3 mg/ml) 0.1 mg/kg rapid IVP/IO (repeat)	0.05 ml	0.1 ml	0.2 ml	0.3 ml	0.5 ml	0.7 ml	0.8 ml	1 ml	1.2 ml	1.3 ml	1.5 ml
0.2 mg/kg rapid IVP/IO (initial)	0.1 ml	0.2 ml	0.35 ml	0.7 ml	1 ml	1.3 ml	1.7 ml	2 ml	2.3 ml	2.6 ml	3 ml
Amiodarone (50 mg/ml) 5 mg/kg IV/IO	0.15 ml	0.35 ml	0.7 ml	1 ml	1.5 ml	2 ml	2.5 ml	3 ml	3.5 ml	4 ml	4.5 ml
Atropine 0.1 mg/ml 0.02 mg/kg IV, IO	1 ml	1 ml	1.4 ml	2 ml	3 ml	4 ml	5 ml	6 ml	7 ml	8 ml	9 ml
CaCl 10% (100 mg/ml) 20 mg/kg slow IV/IO	0.3 ml	0.7 ml	1.4 ml	2 ml	3 ml	4 ml	5 ml	6 ml	7 ml	8 ml	9 ml
Cefotaxime (250 mg/ml) 50 mg/kg IV/IO/IM	0.3 ml	0.7 ml	1.4 ml	2 ml	3 ml	4 ml	5 ml	6 ml	7 ml	8 ml	9 ml
Ceftriaxone (100 mg/ml) 50-100 mg/kg IV/IO/IM	0.75-1.5 ml	1.75-3.5 ml	3.5-7 ml	5-10 ml	7.5-15 ml	10-20 ml	12.5-25 ml	15-30 ml	17.5-35 ml	20-40 ml	22.5-45 ml
Charcoal 1gm/kg PO/NG	n/a	n/a	7 gm	10 gm	15 gm	20 gm	25 gm	30 gm	35 gm	40 gm	45 gm
Dextrose (D50%W) 0.5 gm/kg IV, IO [use D25%W for infant]	3 ml [D25%]	7 ml [D25%]	14 ml [D25%]	20 ml [D25%]	15 ml	20 ml	25 ml	30 ml	35 ml	40 ml	45 ml
Diazepam (5 mg/ml) 0.1-0.2 mg/kg slow IV, IO	0.03-0.06 ml	0.07-0.14 ml	0.14-0.28 ml	0.2-0.4 ml	0.3-0.6 ml	0.4-0.8 ml	0.5-1 ml	0.6-1.2 ml	0.7-1.4 ml	0.8-1.6 ml	0.9-1.8 ml
Diphenhydramine (50 mg/ml) 1 mg/kg IV/IO/IM	n/a	n/a	0.14 ml	0.2 ml	0.3 ml	0.4 ml	0.5 ml	0.6 ml	0.7 ml	0.8 ml	0.9 ml
Epi 1:10,000 0.01 mg/kg IV IO	0.15 ml	0.35 ml	0.7 ml	1 ml	1.5 ml	2 ml	2.5 ml	3 ml	3.5 ml	4 ml	4.5 ml
ET Epinephrine 1:1000 (1 mg/ml) 0.1 mg/kg ET (& 2nd dose IV/IO)	0.15 ml	0.35 ml	0.7 ml	1 ml	1.5 ml	2 ml	2.5 ml	3 ml	3.5 ml	4 ml	4.5 ml

Age	Preterm	Term	6 mos	1 yr	3 yrs	6 yrs	8 yrs	10 yrs	11 yrs	12 yrs	14 yrs
Fosphenytoin 20 mg/kg IV, IM	0.6 ml	1.4 ml	2.8 ml	4 ml	6 ml	8 ml	10 ml	12 ml	14 ml	16 ml	18 ml
Furosemide (10 mg/ml) 1mg/kg slow IV/IO	0.15 ml	0.35 ml	0.7 ml	1 ml	1.5 ml	2 ml	2.5 ml	3 ml	3.5 ml	4 ml	4.5 ml
Lidocaine 2% (20 mg/ml) 1 mg/kg IV, IO	0.08 ml	0.18 ml	0.35 ml	0.5 ml	0.75 ml	1 ml	1.25 ml	1.5 ml	1.75 ml	2 ml	2.25 ml
Methylprednisolone (40 mg/ml) 2 mg/kg IV/IO/IM	0.08 ml	0.18 ml	0.35 ml	0.5 ml	0.75 ml	1 ml	1.25 ml	1.5 ml	1.75 ml	2 ml	2.25 ml
Morphine (1 mg/ml) 0.1 mg/kg IV/IO/IM	0.15 ml	0.35 ml	0.07 ml	1 ml	1.5 ml	2 ml	2.5 ml	3 ml	3.5 ml	4 ml	4.5 ml
NaHCO₃ 8.4% 1 mEq/kg IV, IO [Use 4.2% in neonates]	3 ml [4.2%]	7 ml [4.2%]	7 ml	10 ml	15 ml	20 ml	25 ml	30 ml	35 ml	40 ml	45 ml
Naloxone (1 mg/ml) 0.1 mg/kg IV, IM, SQ	0.15 ml	0.35 ml	0.7 ml	1 ml	1.5 ml	2 ml	2 ml	2 ml	2 ml	2 ml	2 ml
Phenobarbital (65 mg/ml) 10-20 mg/kg slow IV/IO/IM	0.25-0.5 ml	0.4-0.8 ml	1-2 ml	1.5-3 ml	2.3-4.6 ml	3-6 ml	4-8 ml	4.5-9 ml	5.5-11 ml	6-12 ml	7-14 ml
Etomidate (2 mg/ml) 0.3 mg/kg	0.2 ml	0.5 ml	1 ml	1.5 ml	2.3 ml	3 ml	3.75 ml	4.5 ml	5.25 ml	6 ml	6.75 ml
Midazolam (5 mg/ml) 0.1-0.2 mg/kg IV/IM	0.03-0.05 ml	0.07-0.14 ml	0.14-0.28 ml	0.2-0.4 ml	0.3-0.6 ml	0.4-0.8 ml	0.5-1 ml	0.6-1.2 ml	0.7-1.4 ml	0.8-1.6 ml	0.9-1.8 ml
Succinylcholine (20 mg/ml) 1-1.5 mg/kg IV/IO [Infant: 2 mg/kg]	0.15 ml 2 mg/kg	0.35 ml 2 mg/kg	0.7 ml 2 mg/kg	1 ml 2 mg/kg	0.75-1 ml	1-1.5 ml	1.25-1.9 ml	1.5-2.3 ml	1.75-2.6 ml	2 - 3 ml	2.25-3.4 ml
Vecuronium (1 mg/ml) 0.1-0.2 mg/kg IV/IM	0.15-03 ml	0.35-0.7 ml	0.7-0.14 ml	1-2 ml	1.5-3.0 ml	2-4 ml	2.5-5 ml	3-6 ml	3.5-7 ml	4-8 ml	4.5-9 ml

Peds

AMINOPHYLLINE (use 25 mg/ml solution) Loading Dose: 5 mg/kg (0.2 ml/kg in 100 ml D5W over 20–30 minutes. Maintenance Dose: 0.5–1 mg/kg/hour. To mix: add 125 mg to 250 ml D5W (or 50 mg in 100 ml D5W. 1 microdrop/kg/minute of this solution=0.5 mg/kg/hour.

DOBUTAMINE (use 12.5 mg/ml solution) Dose: 2–20 mcg/kg/minute. To mix: add 30 mg (2.4 ml) to 250 ml D5W. 1 microdrop/kg/minute of this solution=2 mcg/kg/minute.

DOPAMINE (use 40 mg/ml solution) Dose: 2–20 mcg/kg/minute. To mix: add 75 mg (1.9 ml) to 250 ml D5W. 1 microdrop/kg/minute of this solution=5 mcg/kg/minute.

EPINEPHRINE (use 1:1000 solution, 1 mg/ml) Dose: 0.1–1 mcg/kg/minute. To mix: add 1.5 mg (1.5 ml) to 250 ml D5W. 1 microdrop/kg/minute of this solution=0.1 mcg/kg/minute.

INAMRINONE (use 5 mg/ml solution) Loading Dose: 0.75 - 1 mg/kg (0.15-0.2 ml/kg) over 10 minutes. Maintenance Dose: 2–20 mcg/kg/min. To mix: add 30 mg (6 ml) to 250 ml NS. 1 microdrop/kg/minute of this solution= 2 mcg/kg/minute.

LIDOCAINE Drip (use 2% solution, 20 mg/ml) Dose: 20–50 mcg/kg/minute. To mix: add 300 mg (15 ml) to 250 ml D5W. 1 microdrop/kg/minute of this solution=20 mcg/kg/minute.

NITROPRUSSIDE (reconstitute 50 mg with 5 ml D5W) Dose: 1-8 mcg/kg/minute. To mix: add 15 mg (1.5 ml) to 250 ml D5W. 1 microdrop/kg/minute of this solution=0.5 mcg/kg/minute.

(for pediatric measurement purposes, this book is appx 10" when opened)

Pediatric Trauma Score—*See page 15*

Intraosseous Infusion

(Most medications, blood products, or solutions that can be given IV, can be given IO)

1 Locate anterior medial (flat) surface of tibia, 2 cm below tibial tuberosity, below growth plate (other sites: distal anterior femur, medial malleolus, iliac crest).

2 Prep area with iodine

3 Advance IO needle at 90° angle through skin, fascia, & bone with constant pressure and twisting motion. Direct needle slightly inferiorly away from epiphyseal plate.

4 A popping sensation will occur (& a lack of resistance) when you have reached the marrow space

5 Attempt to aspirate marrow (you may not get marrow)

6 Infuse fluids and check for infiltration. (D/C if site becomes infiltrated with fluid or medications; apply manual pressure followed by a pressure dressing.)

7 Secure IO needle, tape in place and attach to IV pump

medial malleolus

Pediatric Emergencies—
General Assessment

Airway: Look for obstruction, drooling, trauma.
Breathing: Retractions? Respiratory rate? Good air movement?
Circulation: heart rate? Capillary refill?

Bradycardia means hypoxia. Ventilate!

Mental Status: is child acting normally?

Get History: of present illness / onset, intake, GI habits.
Perform Exam: Fever? Skin color? Other findings?
✛—Kids in shock need aggressive treatment.
• Ventilate. Reassess the airway, especially during transport.
• IV fluid challenge (20cc/kg—repeat if necessary). Don't wait for BP to drop—hypotension is a late sign.
• Rapid transport to a pediatric intensive care facility.
Not every seizure with fever is a febrile seizure

✓**Consider meningitis, especially in children < 2 y.o. (check for a rash that doesn't blanch).**
✓**Early signs of sepsis are subtle: grunting respirations, temperature instability, hypoglycemia, poor feeding, etc.**

Croup

HX—Hx of a cold or flu which develops into a **"barking cough"** at night. Relatively slow onset. Low fever.
✚—Cool, moist air; contact OLMC regarding transport.
Caution—Don't examine the upper airway.

Epiglottitis

HX—Hx of a cold or flu which develops into a high fever at night. **Drooling, difficulty swallowing**, relatively rapid onset. Inspiratory stridor may be present in severe cases.
✚—Cool, moist air. If airway is completely obstructed, ventilate with BVM & O_2
Caution—Don't examine the upper airway. This may cause total airway obstruction.

Croup vs. Epiglottitis

	CROUP	EPIGLOTTITIS
Age	< 3 years old	2 – 6 years old
Sex	♂ > ♀	Both ♂ & ♀
Onset	Gradual (at night)	Relatively rapid
Infection	Viral	Bacterial (H Influenza Type b)
Fever	Low grade	High fever
Breathing	Retractions	Tripod: sitting, leaning forward
Sounds	"Barking cough"	Inspiratory stridor
Voice	Hoarseness	Muffled voice
Other S/ Sx		Drooling, Painful swallowing
Treatment	Fluids, Cool mist, Nebulized Rx, steroids, racemic epi? Observe 6h	O_2, Position of comfort, Avoid agitation, Prepare for intubation (try BVM+ O_2 first) Do not examine airway.

Common Lab Values

(Adult – blood, plasma, or serum)

NOTE: Normal values may vary, depending on the lab or methods used.

Acetone: 0.3–2 mg%
Alcohol (ETOH): 0 mg %; Coma: $\geq$ 400–500 mg%.
Ammonia: 40–70 mcg %
Amylase: 4–25 U/ml, or 80–180 Somogyi units/100 ml
Bicarbonate (HCO3-): 23–29 mEq/L
Bilirubin, direct: 0.1–0.4 mg% (total: 0.3–1.1 mg%)
Calcium: 4.5–5.5 mEq/L. (8.5–11 mg%)
Chloride: 98–109 mEq/L
CO (carbon monoxide): symptoms at 10% saturation
CO_2 content: 24–30 mEq/L; Infants: 20–26 mEq/L
Creatine phosphokinase (CPK): M: 5-35 U/ml; F: 5-25 U/ml
Creatinine: 0.7–1.4 mg%
Fibrinogen (plasma): 200–400 mg%
Glucose (fasting): 65–110 mg %. Diuresis: $\geq$ 180 mg%
Hematocrit: M: 47% (40–50%); F: 42% (37–47%)
Hemoglobin (Hgb): M: 14–18 gm%; F: 12–16 gm%; Child: 12–14 gm%; Newborn: 15–25 gm%.
Iron: 75–175 mg% (less in females)
Lactic dehydrogenase (LDH): 132–240 U/L
Lead: 0–50 mcg%
Lithium: 0.5–1.5 mEq/L (toxicity $\geq$ 2 mEq/L)
Magnesium: 1.5–2.5 mEq/L (1.8–3.0 mg%)
pCO_2 (arterial): 35–45 torr   Newborn: 35–40 torr
pH (arterial): 7.35–7.45 (mean: 7.40)
Platelets: 150,000–350,000 / cu mm.
pO_2 (arterial): 75–100 torr [avg – room air at sea level]
Potassium: 3.5–5.0 mEq/L (14–20 mg%)
Protein: total = 6.0–8.4 gm%
Salicylate: toxicity = $\geq$ 30 mg%
Sodium: 136–147 mEq/L (313–334 mg%)
Transaminase (SGOT): 9–41 U/L
Urea nitrogen (BUN): 6–23 mg%
Urine (specific gravity): 1.003–1.030
WBC (leukocytes): 5,000–10,000 / cu mm.

Phone Numbers	
911 Comm. Center	
American Red Cross	
Chemtrec Emergency	1-800-424-9300
Chemtrec Non-emergency	1-800-262-8200
Child Protective Services	
CISD Team	
Crisis Center	
Domestic Violence Shelter	
HazMat Team	
Homeless Shelter	
Medical Examiner/Coroner	
Medical Resource Center	
National Response Center	1-800-424-8802
Organ Donation Center	
Poison Control Center	
Public Health Department	
Sexual Abuse Hotline	
State /County EMS Office	
Translation Services	
Trauma Center	
Other	
Other	
Other	
Other	
Other	
Other	
Other	
Other	
Other	

Spanish Translations

History & Examination

English	Spanish
I am a paramedic (firefighter; nurse; doctor).	Soy paramédico (bombero; enfermera, enfermero; médico).
I speak a little Spanish.	Hablo un poco de Español.
Is there someone here that speaks English?	¿Hay alguien aquí que habla inglés?
What is your name?	¿Cómo te llamas?
I don't understand.	No entiendo.
Can you speak more slowly please?	¿Por favor, puede hablar más despacio?
Wake up sir/madam.	Despiértate, señor / señora.
Sit up.	Siéntate por favor.
Listen.	Escúchame.
How are you?	¿Cómo estás?
Do you have neck or back pain?	¿Te duele el cuello o la espalda?
Were you unconscious?	Estuviste inconsciente?
Move your fingers and toes.	Mueva los dedos de las manos y los pies.
What day is today?	¿Qué día es hoy?
Where is this?	¿Dónde está?
Where are you?	¿Dónde estás?
What is your telephone number? ...address?	¿Cuál es tu número de teléfono? ...domicilio?
When were you born?	¿Cuando naciste?
Sit here please.	Siéntate aquí, por favor.
Lie down please.	Acuéstate, por favor.
Do you have pain?	¿Tienes dolor?
...trouble breathing?	...dificultad para respirar?
...weakness?	...débilidad?
Where?	¿Dónde?
Show me where it hurts with your hand.	Muéstrame con tu mano dónde te duele.
Does the pain increase when you breathe?	¿Te aumenta el dolor cuando respiras?
Breathe deeply through your mouth. ...Breathe slowly.	Respira profundo por la boca. ...Respira despacio.
What medicines do you take?	¿Qué medicinas tómas?
Have you been drinking?	¿Has estado tomado alcohol?
Have you taken any drugs?	¿Has tomado alguna droga?

124

Do you have chest pain?	¿Tienes dolor de pecho?
...heart problems?	problemas de corazón?
...diabetes?	diabétes?
...asthma?	asma?
...allergies?	alergias?
Have you had this pain before?	¿En otra ocasión has tenido este dolor?
How long ago?	¿Hace cúanto tiempo?
Are you sick to your stomach?	¿Tienes nausea o asco?
Are you pregnant?	¿Estás embarazada?
Do you need to vomit?	¿Necesitas vomitar?
You will be OK.	Todo estará bien.
It's not serious.	No es serio.
It is serious.	Es serio.

Treatment

Please don't move.	Por favor, no te muevas.
What's the matter?	¿Qué pasa?
Do you want to go to the hospital?	¿Quieres ir al hospital?
To which hospital?	¿A cuál hospital?
You must go to the hospital.	Tienes que ir al hospital.
We're going to take you to the hospital.	Te vamos a llevar al hospital.
We are going to give you oxygen.	Te vamos a dar oxígeno
We are going to apply a C-collar.	Te vamos a poner un collarín.
We are going to give you an IV.	Te vamos a poner un suero.

Miscellaneous

Thank you.	Gracias.	lungs	los pulmónes
hand	la mano	arm	el brazo
Excuse me.	Perdóname	meds	medicinas
head	la cabeza	back	la espalda
Hello	Hola	mouth	la boca
heart	el corazón	fracture	una fractura
Goodbye	Adiós	neck	el cuello
to help	ayudar	cancer	cáncer
Yes	Sí	penis	el pene
foot	el pie	chest	el pecho
No	No	wrist	la muñeca
hypertension	presión alta	drugs	droga
abdomen	el abdomen	stroke	ataque
leg	la pierna	ear	el oído
ankle	el tobillo	eye	el ojo
vagina	la vagina	throat	la garganta

Prescription Drugs

A

ABILIFY (aripiprazole): psychotropic, Rx: schizophrenia
Acarbose (PRECOSE): oral hypoglycemic, Rx: diabetes
ACCOMPLIA (rimonabant): cannabinoid receptor blocker, Rx: obesity, smoking cessation
ACCOLATE (zafirlukast): bronchospasm inhibitor, Rx: asthma
ACCUNEB (albuterol): beta-2 bronchodilator, Rx: asthma, COPD
ACCUPRIL (quinapril): ACE inhibitor, Rx: HTN, CHF
ACCURETIC (quinapril, HCTZ): ACE inhibitor, diuretic, Rx: HTN
ACCUTANE (isotretinoin): Rx: severe cystic acne
Acebutolol (SECTRAL): ß-blocker, Rx: HTN, angina, arrhythmias
ACEON (perindopril): ACE inhibitor, Rx: HTN
Acetaminophen (TYLENOL): non-narcotic analgesic
Acetazolamide (DIAMOX): diuretic / anticonvulsant, Rx: glaucoma, CHF, epilepsy, mountain sickness
Acetylcysteine (MUCOSIL): mucolytic, Rx: asthma
ACIPHEX (rabeprazole): inhibits gastric acid secretion, Rx: ulcers
ACLOVATE (alclometasone): steroid anti-inflammatory
Acrivastine (SEMPREX-D): antihistamine / decongestant
ACTICIN CREAM (permethrin): scabicide, Rx: scabies
ACTIFED (triprolidine + pseudoephedrine): antihistamine / decongestant, Rx: allergies
ACTIGALL (ursodiol): bile acid, Rx: gallstones
ACTIQ (fentanyl): oral transmucosal narcotic analgesic, Rx: CA
ACTIVELLA (estradiol, norethindrone): hormones, Rx: menopause
ACTOS (pioglitazone): oral hypoglycemic, Rx: diabetes
ACULAR (ketorolac): NSAID analgesic, Rx: allergic conjunctivitis
Acyclovir (ZOVIRAX): antiviral, Rx: herpes, shingles, chicken pox
ADALAT, ADALAT CC (nifedipine): Ca++ blocker, Rx: angina, HTN
Adapalene (DIFFERIN): anti-acne, Rx: acne vulgaris
ADDERALL (amphetamines): CNS stimulant, Rx: ADD
ADIPEX-P (phentermine): appetite suppressant / stimulant
ADOXA (doxycycline): an antibiotic

ADRENALIN (epinephrine): bronchodilator, Rx: asthma
ADVAIR DISKUS (fluticasone, salmeterol): steroid antiinflammatory, beta-2 bronchodilator, Rx: asthma, COPD
ADVICOR (niacin, lovastatin): vasodilator, cholesterol reducer
ADVIL (ibuprofen): NSAID analgesic
AEROBID, AEROBID M (flunisolide): steroid anti-inflammatory inhaler, Rx: asthma, bronchitis
AEROLATE, AEROLATE III, AEROLATE Jr., (theophylline): xanthine bronchodilator, Rx: asthma, COPD
AGENERASE (amprenavir): antiretroviral agent, Rx: AIDS, HIV
AGGRENOX (aspirin, dipyridamole): antiplatelet agents, Rx: to reduce the risk of stroke
AGRYLIN (anagrelide): reduces platelet #s, Rx: thrombocythemia
AKINETON (biperiden): antiparkinsonian, Rx: prophylaxis of EPS
ALAMAST (pemirolast): anti-inflammatory, Rx: allergic conjunctivitis
Albendazole (ALBENZA): anthelmintic, Rx: tapeworm
ALBENZA (albendazole): anthelmintic, Rx: tapeworm
Albuterol (PROVENTIL): ß-2 bronchodilator, Rx: asthma, COPD
ALDACTAZIDE (HCTZ, spironolactone): diuretics, Rx: HTN
ALDACTONE (spironolactone): potassium-sparing diuretic
ALDARA (Imiquimod): immune modifier, Rx: genital warts
ALDOCHLOR (methyldopa + chlorothiazide): antihypertensive / diuretic
ALDOMET (methyldopa): an antihypertensive
ALDORIL (methyldopa + HCTZ): antihypertensive compound
ALESSE, ALESSE 28 (levonorgestrel, estradiol): oral contraceptive
ALEVE (naproxen): NSAID analgesic
ALLEGRA (fexofenadine): antihistamine, Rx: allergies
Allopurinol (ZYLOPRIM): reduces serum uric acid, Rx: gout
ALORA (estradiol): hormone, Rx: menopause
Alosetron (LOTRONEX): antidiarrheal, Rx: irritable bowel synd.
Alprazolam (XANAX): benzodiazepine hypnotic
ALTACE (ramipril): ACE inhibitor, Rx: hypertension
ALTOCOR (lovastatin): cholesterol reducer
ALTOPREV (lovastatin): statin, cholesterol reducer
ALUPENT (metaproterenol): ß-2 bronchodilator, Rx: asthma
Amantadine (SYMMETREL): antiviral, antiparkinsonian, Rx: influenza A, extrapyramidal symptoms

AMARYL (glimepiride): oral hypoglycemic, Rx: diabetes mellitus

AMBIEN (zolpidem): hypnotic, Rx: insomnia

AMBISOME (amphotericin B): antifungal, Rx: fungal infections

Amcinonide (CYCLOCORT): steroid anti-inflammatory, Rx: pruritus, inflammation

AMERGE (naratriptan): antimigraine, Rx: acute migraine HA

AMEVIVE (alefacept): immunosuppressive protein, Rx: psoriasis

Amikacin (AMIKIN): antibiotic, Rx: infections

AMIKIN (amikacin): an antibiotic

Amiloride (MIDAMOR): diuretic, Rx: CHF, hypertension

Aminobenzoate (POTABA): antifibrotic, Rx: scleroderma, Peyronie's disease

Aminophylline : bronchodilator, Rx: COPD, asthma

Aminosalicylic Acid (PASER): antibacterial, Rx: tuberculosis

Amiodarone (CORDARONE): antiarrhythmic, Rx: arrhythmias

Amitriptyline: a tricyclic antidepressant

AMITRIZA (lubiprostone): intestinal stimulant, Rx: chronic idiopathic constipation

Amlodipine (LOTREL): calcium blocker, Rx: HTN, angina

Amoxapine (ASENDIN): tricyclic antidepressant

Amoxicillin (AMOXIL): an antibiotic

AMOXIL (amoxicillin): an antibiotic

Amphetamine (ADDERALL): stimulant, Rx: ADHD

Amphotericin B (FUNGIZONE): an antifungal agent

Ampicillin (omnipen): antibiotic

Amprenavir (AGENERASE): antiretroviral, Rx: AIDS, HIV

Amylase (ARCO-LASE): digestive enzyme, Rx: GI disorders

ANADROL-50 (oxymetholone): anabolic steroid / androgen, Rx: anemia

ANAFRANIL (clomipramine): tricyclic antidepressant

ANALPRAM HC (pramoxine): topical anesthetic, Rx: itching, pain

ANAPROX, ANAPROX DS (naproxen): NSAID analgesic / anti-inflammatory agent

Anastrozole (ARIMIDEX): estrogen inhibitor, antineoplastic, Rx: breast cancer

ANCOBON (flucytosine): an antifungal agent

ANDRODERM (testosterone): androgen / steroid / masculinizing hormone, Rx: hypogonadism, delayed puberty

ANEXSIA (hydrocodone, APAP): narcotic analgesic compound

ANOLOR 300 (butalbital, acetaminophen, caffeine): sedative, analgesic, Rx: pain relief

ANTABUSE (disulfiram): inhibits metabolism of alcohol, Rx: alcohol addiction

Anthralin (MICANOL): antipsoriatic, hair growth stimulant, Rx: psoriasis, alopecia

ANTIVERT (meclizine): antinauseant, Rx: vertigo

ANZEMET (dolasetron): antinauseant, antiemetic, Rx: chemotherapy, nausea & vomiting

APAP (acetaminophen): a non-narcotic analgesic

APHRODYNE (yohimbine): alpha blocker, Rx: impotence

APOKYN (apomorphine): dopamine antagonist, Rx Parkinson's disease

APRI (desogrestel, ethinyl estradiol): oral contraceptive

AQUAMEPHYTON (phytonadione): vitamin K, antihemorrhagic, Rx: blood coagulation disorders

ARALEN (chloroquine): an antimalarial agent

ARANESP (darbepoetin): increases RBC production, Rx: anemia, renal failure, chemotherapy

ARAVA (leflunomide): antiarthritic, anti-inflammatory, Rx: rheumatoid arthritis

ARCO-LASE PLUS (digestive enzymes, hyoscyamine, atropine, phenobarbital): Rx: poor digestion

ARICEPT (donepezil): cholinergic enhancer, Rx: Alzheimer's

ARIMIDEX (anastrozole): estrogen inhibitor, antineoplastic, Rx: breast cancer

ARISTOCORT (triamcinolone): steroid anti-inflammatory

ARMOUR THYROID thyroid hormone

ARTHROTEC (diclofenac, misoprostol): NSAID analgesic, antiulcer, Rx: arthritis

ASA (acetylsalicylic acid): aspirin, a NSAID analgesic

ASACOL (mesalamine): anti-inflammatory agent, Rx: colitis

Ascorbic acid Vitamin C

ASTELIN (azelastine): antihistamine, Rx: allergic rhinitis

ASTRAMORPH PF (morphine): narcotic analgesic

ATACAND (candesartan): antihypertensive, Rx: hypertension

ATARAX (hydroxyzine): sedative / tranquilizer / antihistamine, Rx: urticaria, anxiety

Atenolol (TENORMIN): beta blocker, Rx: HTN, arrhythmias

Atenolol & Chlorthalidone: ß-blocker, diuretic, Rx: HTN

ATIVAN (lorazepam): a benzodiazepine hypnotic

Atovaquone (MEPRON): antiprotozoal, Rx: pneumonia

ATRIPLA (tenofovir, emtricitabine, efavirenz): antivirals, Rx: HIV / AIDS

ATROVENT (ipratropium): anticholinergic bronchodilator, Rx: COPD

AUGMENTIN (amoxicillin, clavulanate potassium): an antibiotic

AVALIDE (irbesartan, hydrochlorothiazide): antihypertensive compound, Rx: hypertension

AVANDAMET (rosiglitazone, metformin): oral hypoglycemics, Rx: diabetes

AVANDIA (rosiglitazone): oral hypoglycemic, Rx: diabetes

AVAPRO (irbesartan): antihypertensive, Rx: hypertension

AVELOX (moxifloxacin): antibiotic, Rx: bronchitis, pneumonia

AVIANE (levonorgestrel, ethinyl estradiol): oral contraceptive

AVINZA (morphine): narcotic analgesic, Rx: severe pain

AVONEX (interferon): antiviral, Rx: MS

AXERT (almotriptan): antimigraine, Rx: migraine headaches

AXID (nizatadine): histamine-2 antagonist, which inhibits gastric acid secretion, Rx: ulcers

AYGESTIN (norethindrone): hormone, Rx: amenorrhea, endometriosis

AZACTAM (aztreonam): antibiotic, Rx: UTI, infections

AZASAN (azathioprine): immunosupressant, Rx: rheumatoid arthritis, prevents kidney transplant rejection

Azathioprine (IMURAN): immunosuppressant, Rx: organ transplants, arthritis

Azelaic Acid (AZELEX): antimicrobial, Rx: acne

Azelastine (OPTIVAR): antihistamine, anti-inflammatory, Rx: allergic conjunctivitis

Azithromycin (ZITHROMAX): antibiotic

AZMACORT (triamcinolone): steroid anti-inflammatory, Rx: asthma, bronchitis

AZOPT OPTH (brinzolamide): reduces intraocular pressure, Rx: glaucoma, ocular hypertension

AZT (zidovudine): an antiviral agent, Rx: HIV (AIDS) virus

AZULFIDINE-EN (sulfasalazine): anti-infective, anti-inflammatory, Rx: colitis, arthritis

B

B & O SUPPRETTES (belladonna, opium): narcotic analgesic, antispasmodic, Rx: pain relief

Bacitracin (bacitracin): antibiotic, Rx: pneumonia, staphylococci infection

Baclofen: muscle relaxant, Rx: MS, spinal cord disease

BACTROBAN (mupirocin): topical antibacterial, Rx: skin infection

Balsalazide (COLAZAL): anti-inflammatory, Rx: ulcerative colitis

Beclomethasone (BECONASE): steroid anti-inflammatory

BECONASE AQ (beclomethasone): steroid anti-inflammatory

Belladonna (BELLADENAL): antispasmodic, Rx: irritable bowel syndrome
BENEMID (probenecid): uricosuric, Rx: gout
Benicar (olmesartan): angiotensin II blocker, Rx: HTN
BENTYL (dicyclomine): GI tract antispasmodic
Benzoic Acid (PROSED DS): antibacterial, antifungal, Rx: urinary tract pain, cystitis, urethritis
Benzonatate (TESSALON): non-narcotic antitussive, Rx: cough
Benzoyl Peroxide (PANOXYL): antibacterial, Rx: acne
Benztropine (COGENTIN): anticholinergic, Rx: Parkinson's disease
Betamethasone (CELESTONE): steroid anti-inflammatory
BETAPACE (sotalol): ß-blocker, Rx: angina, HTN, arrhythmias
BETASERON (interferon): immunologic, Rx Multiple Sclerosis
Betaxolol (KERLONE): ß-blocker, Rx: HTN
Bethanechol (URECHOLINE): vagomimetic, increases bladder tone, Rx: urinary retention
BETOPTIC (betaxolol): ß-1 blocker eyedrops, Rx: glaucoma
BEXTRA (valdecoxib): COX-2 inhibitor, Rx: arthritis, dysmenorrhea
BIAXIN (clarithromycin) an antibiotic
Bicalutamide (CASODEX): antiandrogen, Rx: prostate cancer
BICILLIN (penicillin): an antibiotic
BIDIL (hydralazine, isosorbide dinitrate): antihypertensive, vasodilator, Rx: heart failure
BILTRICIDE (praziquantel): anthelmintic, Rx: schistosomiasis, flukes
Biperiden (AKINETON): anticholinergic, Rx: Parkinson's disease, EPS
Bisacodyl (DULCOLAX): laxative, Rx: constipation
Bisoprolol (ZEBETA): ß-blocker, Rx: HTN
Bisoprolol / HCTZ: ß-blocker, diuretic, Rx: HTN
Bitolterol (TORNALATE): ß-bronchodilator, Rx: asthma
BLEPHAMIDE (sulfacetamide, prednisolone): antibacterial, steroid anti-inflammatory, Rx: ocular infections
BLOCADREN (timolol): ß-blocker, Rx: angina, HTN, arrhythmias
BONIVA (ibandronate): osteoclast inhibitor, Rx: osteoporosis prophylaxis
BONTRIL PDM, BONTRIL Slow Release (phendimetrazine): stimulant, appetite suppressant, Rx: obesity
BRETHINE (terbutaline): ß-2 bronchodilator, Rx: COPD, asthma
BREVICON: an oral contraceptive

Brimonidine (ALPHAGAN): alpha agonist, lowers intraocular pressure, Rx: glaucoma

Brinzolamide (AZOPT OPHTHALMIC): reduces intraocular pressure, Rx: glaucoma, ocular hypertension

Bromocriptine (PARLODEL): ergot, Rx: Parkinson's disease, hypogonadism, infertility, amenorrhea

Brompheniramine (BROMFED): antihistamine, Rx: allergies

Budesonide (RHINOCORT): corticosteroid, Rx: allergic rhinitis

Bumetanide (BUMEX): diuretic, Rx: edema, CHF

BUPAP (butalbital, acetaminophen): sedative/analgesic, Rx: H/A

BUPRENEX (buprenorphine): narcotic analgesic

Buprenorphine (BUPRENEX): narcotic analgesic

Bupropion (WELLBUTRIN): an antidepressant

BuSpar (buspirone): antianxiety agent, Rx: anxiety disorders

Buspirone (busPRIone): antianxiety agent, Rx: anxiety disorders

BusPRIone (buspirone): antianxiety agent, Rx: anxiety disorders

Busulfan (MYLERAN): anticancer agent, Rx: leukemia

Butabarbital (PYRIDIUM): barbiturate sedative / antispasmodic

Butalbital (FIORINAL): barbiturate muscle relaxant / sedative

Butalbital, Acetaminophen, Caffeine: sedative / analgesic

Butoconazole (GYNAZOLE-1): antifungal, Rx: yeast infections

Butorphanol (STADOL): narcotic analgesic

BYETTA (exenatide): increases insulin release, Rx: diabetes

C

CALAN, CALAN SR (verapamil): calcium blocker, Rx: angina, hypertension, PSVT prophylaxis, headache

Calcifediol (CALDEROL): vitamin D supplement, Rx: hypocalcemia, bone disease

CALCIFEROL (ergocalciferol): vitamin D, Rx: hypocalcemia, hypoparathyroidism, rickets, osteodystrophy

CALCIJEX (calcitriol): vitamin D supplement, Rx: hypocalcemia, hypoparathyroidism, bone disease

Calcipotriene (DOVONEX): vitamin D, Rx: psoriasis

Calcitonin-Salmon (MIACALCIN): bone resorption inhibitor hormone, Rx: hypercalcemia, Paget's disease, osteoporosis

Calcitriol (ROCALTROL): vitamin D supplement, Rx: hypocalcemia, hypoparathyroidism, bone disease

CAMILA (norethindrone): oral contraceptive

CAMPRAL (acamprosate): reduces withdrawal symptoms, Rx: alcohol abstinence

CANASA (mesalamine): anti-inflammatory, Rx: ulcerative proctitis
Candesartan Cilexetil (ATACAND): angiotensin II antagonist antihypertensive, Rx: HTN
CAPITAL w/ Codeine (APAP, codeine): narcotic analgesic
Captopril (CAPOTEN): ACE inhibitor, Rx: HTN, CHF
CARAFATE (sucralfate): an anti ulcer agent
Carbamazepine (TEGRETOL): an anticonvulsant, Rx: epilepsy
CARBATROL (carbamazepine): anticonvulsant, analgesic, Rx: epilepsy, trigeminal neuralgia
Carbenicillin (GEOCILLIN): antibiotic, Rx: UTI
Carbetapentane (RYNATUSS): antitussive, Rx: coughs
Carbidopa & Levodopa (SINEMET): dopamine precursors, Rx: Parkinson's Disease
CARDIZEM LA (diltiazem): Ca++ blocker, Rx: angina, HTN, PSVT
CARDURA (doxazosin): alpha blocker, Rx: HTN, prostatic hypertrophy
Carisoprodol (SOMA): muscle relaxant / analgesic
Carvedilol (COREG): beta & alpha blocker, Rx: angina, heart failure, HTN
Caspofungin (CANCIDAS): antifungal antibiotic, Rx: fungal infection
CATAFLAM (diclofenac): NSAID analgesic
CATAPRES, CATAPRES TTS (clonidine): an antihypertensive
CAUDET (amlodipine, atorvastatin): calcium blocker, lipid lowering agent, Rx: HTN & high cholesterol
CECLOR (cefaclor): an antibiotic
CEDAX (ceftibuten): an antibiotic
Cefaclor (CECLOR): antibiotic
Cefadroxil (DURICEF): an antibiotic
Cefazolin (ANCEF): an antibiotic
Cefdinir (OMNICEF): antibiotic, Rx: infections
Cefixime (SUPRAX): broad spectrum antibiotic
CEFIZOX (ceftizomine): antibiotic, Rx: infections
CEFOBID (cefoperazone): antibiotic, Rx: respiratory tract infections
Cefoperazone (CEFOBID): antibiotic, Rx: respiratory tract infections
Cefotaxime (CLAFORAN): antibiotic, Rx: infections
Cefotetan (CEFOTAN): an antibiotic
Cefoxitin (MEFOXIN): antibiotic, Rx: infections
Cefpodoxime (VANTIN): antibiotic, Rx: infections
Cefprozil (CEFZIL): an antibiotic
Ceftazidime (CEPTAZ): antibiotic, Rx: infections

Ceftibuten (CEDAX): an antibiotic
CEFTIN (cefuroxime): an antibiotic
Ceftizoxime (CEFIZOX): antibiotic, Rx: infections
Ceftriaxone (ROCEPHIN): antibiotic, Rx: infections
Cefuroxime (CEFTIN): antibiotic, Rx: infections
CEFZIL (cefprozil): an antibiotic
CELEBREX (celecoxib): NSAID analgesic, Rx: arthritis
Celecoxib (CELEBREX): NSAID analgesic, Rx: arthritis
CELEXA (citalopram): antidepressant, Rx: depression
CellCept (mycophenolate): immunosuppressant, Rx: organ transplants
CELONTIN (methsuximide): anticonvulsant, Rx: absence Sz
CENESTIN (estrogens): hormone, Rx: menopause
Cephalexin (KEFLEX): an antibiotic
CEREBYX (fosphenytoin): anticonvulsant, Rx: status epilepticus
CEREZYME (imiglucerase): enzyme, Rx: Gauchers disease
CESAMET (nabilone): synthetic cannabinoid, antinauseant, Rx: nausea & vomiting 2° chemotherapy
Cetirizine (ZYRTEC): antihistamine, Rx: allergic rhinitis, urticaria
Cevimeline (EVOXAC): cholinergic, Rx: dry mouth from Sjogren's syndrome
CHIBROXIN (norfloxacin): antibacterial, Rx: conjunctivitis
Chloral Hydrate: a sedative
Chlorambucil (LEUKERAN): alkylating agent, Rx: leukemia, lymphomas, Hodgkin's disease
Chlordiazepoxide (LIBRIUM): a benzodiazepine hypnotic
Chloroquine (ARALEN): antimalarial, amebicidal agent, Rx: malaria
Chlorothiazide (DIURIL): an antihypertensive / diuretic
Chloroxylenol (GORDOCHOM): antifungal, Rx: athlete's foot, ringworm
Chlorpheniramine (NALEXA): antihistamine, Rx: colds, allergies
Chlorpromazine (THORAZINE): a major tranquilizer
Chlorpropamide (DIABINESE): oral hypoglycemic, Rx: diabetes
Chlorthalidone (HYGROTON): antihypertensive / diuretic
Chlorzoxazone (PARAFON FORTE): skeletal muscle relaxant
Cholestyramine (PREVALITE): cholesterol lowering agent
CIALIS (tadalafil): vasodilator, Rx: male erectile dysfunction
Ciclopirox (LOPROX): antifungal, Rx: ringworm, candida
Cidofovir (VISTIDE): antiviral, Rx: cytomegalovirus in AIDS
Cilastatin (PRIMAXIN): antibacterial agent, Rx: infection

Cilostazol (PLETAL): vasodilator, platelet inhibitor, Rx: leg cramps
Cimetidine (TAGAMET): histamine-2 blocker, inhibits gastric acid secretion, Rx: ulcers
CIPRO (ciprofloxacin): an antimicrobial agent
Ciprofloxacin (CIPRO): antibiotic, Rx: infection
Citalopram (CELEXA): antidepressant, Rx: depression
Cladribine (LEUSTATIN): antineoplastic, Rx: leukemia, cancer
CLAFORAN (cefotaxime): an antibiotic
CLARAVIS (isotretinoin): anti-inflammatory, Rx: psoriasis
Clarithromycin (BIAXIN): antibiotic
Clavulanate (AUGMENTIN): antibiotic enhancer, Rx: improves effectiveness of penicillins
CLEOCIN VAGINAL CREAM (clindamycin): antibiotic, Rx: bacterial vaginosis
CLEOCIN, CLEOCIN T (clindamycin): antibiotic, Rx: acne
CLIMARA, CLIMARA PRO (estradiol) hormone, Rx: menopause
Clindamycin (CLEOCIN): an antibiotic
CLINDETS PLEDGETS (clindamycin): antibiotic, Rx: acne
CLINORIL (sulindac): NSAID analgesic, Rx: arthritis
Clobetasol (TEMOVATE): steroid anti-inflammatory, Rx: dermatoses
CLOBEX (clobetasol): steroid anti-inflammatory, Rx: dermatoses
Clofibrate (ATROMID-S): reduces serum lipids
Clomipramine (ANAFRANIL): a tricyclic antidepressant
Clonazepam (KLONOPIN): anticonvulsant, Rx: seizures, panic disorders
Clonidine (CATAPRES): an antihypertensive agent
Clopidogrel (PLAVIX): antiplatelet, Rx: ACS, AMI, stroke
Clorazepate (TRANXENE): antianxiety / anticonvulsant
CLORPRES (clonidine, chlorthalidone): antihypertensive, diuretic, Rx: HTN
Clotrimazole (MYCELEX): antifungal, Rx: candida
Clozapine (CLOZARIL): antipsychotic, Rx: schizophrenia
CLOZARIL (clozapine): psychotropic, Rx: schizophrenia
COCAINE (cocaine HCl): mucous membrane anesthetic
Codeine: a narcotic analgesic / antitussive
COGENTIN (benztropine): an antiparkinsonian, Rx: EPS
COGNEX (tacrine): cholinomimetic / Ach-ase inhibitor, Rx: Alzheimer's Disease
COLACE (docusate): a stool softener
COLAZAL (balsalazide): anti-inflammatory, Rx: ulcerative colitis

Colchicine (ColBENEMID): reduces incidence of gout attacks
Colesevelam (WELCHOL): lowers serum cholesterol, Rx: hyperlipidemia
COLESTID (colestipol): reduces serum cholesterol
Colestipol (COLESTID): reduces serum cholesterol
Colistimethate (COLY-MYCIN M): antibiotic, Rx: pseudomonas infection
Colistin (CORTISPORIN-TC): antibiotic, Rx: ear infections
COLY-MYCIN M (colistimethane): antibiotic, Rx: pseudomonas infection
COMBIPATCH (estradiol, norethindrone): estrogens, Rx: menopause symptoms
COMBIVENT (albuterol, ipratropium): bronchodilators, Rx: asthma
COMBIVIR (lamivudine, zidovudine): antivirals, Rx: HIV, AIDS
COMPAZINE (prochlorperazine): a phenothiazine antiemetic
COMTAN (entacapone): COMT inhibitor, Rx: Parkinson's disease
CONCERTA (methylphenidate): stimulant, Rx: ADHD, narcolepsy
CONDYLOX (podofilox): antimitotic, Rx: anogenital warts
COPAXONE (glatiramer): neurologic agent, Rx: MS
COPEGUS (ribavirin): antiviral, Rx: Hepatitis C
CORDARONE (amiodarone): antiarrhythmic, Rx: VF, VT
CORDRAN (flurandrenolide): steroid anti-inflammatory
CORDYMAX CS4 (cordyceps sinensis): dietary supplement, Rx: fatigue
COREG (carvedilol): ß & alpha blocker, Rx: HTN, CHF, angina
CORMAX (clobetasol): steroid anti-inflammatory, Rx: dermatoses
CORTEF (hydroxycortisone): steroid anti-inflammatory
CORTIC Ear Drops (chloroxylenol, pramoxine, hydrocortisone): antiseptic, antifungal, steroid anti-inflammatory
CORTIFOAM (hydrocortisone): steroid anti-inflammatory, Rx: proctitis
CORTISOL (hydrocortisone): steroid anti-inflammatory
Cortisone (CORTONE): steroid anti-inflammatory
CORTISPORIN (neomycin, polymyxin, hydrocortisone): antibiotic / steroid anti-inflammatory
CORTISPORIN-TC OTIC (neomycin, hydrocortisone): antibiotic, steroid anti-inflammatory, Rx: ear infection
CORTONE (cortisone): steroid anti-inflammatory
CORVERT (ibutilide): antiarrhythmic, Rx: atrial fibrillation, flutter

CORZIDE (bendroflumethiazide, nadolol): ß-blocker, diuretic, Rx: HTN

COSOPT (timolol, dorzolamide): beta-blocker, decreases intraocular pressure, Rx: glaucoma

COUMADIN (warfarin): an anticoagulant, Rx: thrombosis prophylaxis

COVERA HS (verapamil): calcium blocker, Rx: HTN, angina

COZAAR (losartan): an antihypertensive

CREON, CREON 5, CREON 10, CREON 20 (pancrelipase): pancreatic enzyme supplement

CRESTOR (rosuvastatin): statin, cholesterol reducer

CRIXIVAN (indinavir): protease inhibitor antiviral, Rx: AIDS

Cromolyn (INTAL): antiallergenic, Rx: asthma prophylaxis

CRYSELLE (norgestrel, ethinyl estradiol): oral contraceptive

CUPRIMINE (penicillamine): chelating agent, anti-inflammatory, Rx: Wilson's disease, arthritis, heavy metal toxicity

CUTIVATE (fluticasone): topical steroid anti-inflammatory, Rx: dermatoses

Cyanocobalamin (vitamin B-12): Rx: anemia

CYCLESSA (desoxygestrel, estradiol): oral contraceptive

Cyclobenzaprine (FLEXERIL): skeletal muscle relaxant

CYCLOCORT TOPICAL (amcinonide): steroid antiinflammatory, Rx: pruritus, dermatitis

Cyclosporine (SANDIMMUNE): immunosuppressant agent, Rx: prophylaxis of rejection of transplanted organs

CYLERT (pemoline): a stimulant, Rx: ADHD

CYMBALTA (duloxetine): SSRI, Rx: depression, diabetic neuropathy

Cyproheptadine (PERIACTIN): an antihistamine

CYSTOSPAZ, CYSTOSPAZ-M (hyoscyamine): urinary tract antispasmodic

CYTOMEL (liothyronine): thyroid hormone, Rx: hypothyroidism

CYTOTEC (misoprostol): prevents gastric ulcers from NSAIDs

CYTOVENE (ganciclovir): antiviral, Rx: cytomegalovirus, ARC, AIDS

D

d4T stavudine (ZERIT): antiviral, Rx: HIV

ddC (HIVID, zalcitabine): antiviral, Rx: AIDS

DALMANE (flurazepam): anxiolytic, Rx: insomnia

DANTRIUM (dantrolene): skeletal muscle antispasmodic, Rx: multiple sclerosis, cerebral palsy

Dantrolene (DANTRIUM): skeletal muscle antispasmodic, Rx: multiple sclerosis, cerebral palsy

Dapsone: antibacterial drug, Rx: leprosy, dermatitis herpetiformis
DARANIDE (dichlorphenamide): lowers intraocular pressure, Rx: glaucoma
DARAPRIM (pyrimethamine): antiparasitic, Rx: malaria, toxoplasmosis
DARVOCET-N (propoxyphene, APAP): narcotic analgesic
DARVON (propoxyphene): narcotic analgesic
DARVON Compound (propoxyphene, ASA, caffeine) narcotic analgesic compound
DAYPRO (oxaprozin): NSAID, Rx arthritis
DDAVP (desmopressin): antidiuretic hormone, Rx: nocturia, diabetes insipidus
DECADRON (dexamethasone): steroid anti-inflammatory
DECADRON L.A. (dexamethasone): steroid anti-inflammatory
DECLOMYCIN (demeclocycline): an antibiotic
DEFEN-LA (pseudoephedrine, guaifenesin): decongestant, expectorant, Rx: the common cold
Deferoxamine (DESFERAL): iron-chelator, Rx: iron toxicity
Delavirdine (RESCRIPTOR): antiviral, Rx: HIV
Deltasone (prednisone): steroid anti-inflammatory
DEMADEX (torsemide): diuretic, Rx: HTN, edema, CHF, kidney disease, liver disease
Demeclocycline (DECLOMYCIN): an antibiotic, Rx: infections
DEMEROL (meperidine): narcotic analgesic
DEMULEN: oral contraceptive
DENAVIR (penciclovir): antiviral, Rx: herpes, cold sores
DEPACON (divalproex): antiepileptic, Rx: absence seizures
DEPADE (naltrexone): opioid antidote, Rx: narcotic addiction
DEPAKENE (valproic acid): antiepileptic, Rx: epilepsy
DEPAKOTE, DEPAKOTE ER (divalproex): anticonvulsant, antimigraine, Rx: migraine headache, absence seizures
DEPO-MEDROL (methylprednisolone): steroid anti-inflammatory
DEPO-PROVERA (medroxyprogesterone): contraceptive / anticancer agent, Rx: endometrial or renal CA
DEPRENYL (selegiline): MAO inhibitor, Rx: Parkinson's disease
Desipramine (NORPRAMIN): tricyclic antidepressant
Desmopressin (DDAVP): antidiuretic, Rx: bed-wetting, diabetes insipidus
DESOGEN (desogestrel, estradiol): oral contraceptive
Desogestrel (DESOGEN): an oral contraceptive
Desonide (DESOWEN): steroid anti-inflammatory

Desoximetasone (TOPICORT): steroid anti-inflammatory, Rx: dermatitis
DESOXYN (methamphetamine): a stimulant
DETROL (tolterodine): urinary bladder antispasmodic, Rx: overactive bladder
Dexamethasone (DECADRON): steroid anti-inflammatory
DEXEDRINE (dextroamphetamine): a stimulant
Dextroamphetamine (DEXEDRINE): stimulant, Rx: ADHD, narcolepsy
Dextroamphetamine & Amphetamine (ADDERALL): stimulants, Rx: ADHD
DEXTROSTAT (dextroamphetamine): stimulant, Rx: ADHD, narcolepsy
DIABETA (glyburide): oral hypoglycemic, Rx: diabetes
DIABINESE (chlorpropamide): oral hypoglycemic, Rx: diabetes
DIAMOX (acetazolamide): diuretic / anticonvulsant, Rx: glaucoma, CHF, epilepsy, mountain sickness
Diazepam (VALIUM): anxiolytic, Rx: anxiety, Sz, panic disorder
DIBENZYLINE (phenoxybenzamine): alpha blocker, Rx: HTN, sweating
Dichloralphenazone (MIDRIN): sedative, Rx: headaches
Dichlorphenamide (DARANIDE): lowers intraocular pressure, Rx: glaucoma
Diclofenac (VOLTAREN): NSAID, analgesic, Rx: arthritis
Dicyclomine (BENTYL): anticholinergic, Rx: colitis
Didanosine (VIDEX): antiviral, Rx: AIDS, HIV
DIDRONEL (etidronate): bone metabolism regulator, Rx: Paget's disease, total hip replacement
Diethylpropion (TENUATE): stimulant, appetite suppressant, Rx: obesity
Difenoxin (MOTOFEN): antidiarrheal, Rx: diarrhea
DIFFERIN (adapalene): topical retinoid, Rx: acne
Diflorasone (PSORCON): steroid anti-inflammatory, Rx: dermatoses
DIFLUCAN (fluconazole): an antifungal agent
Diflunisal (DOLOBID): NSAID analgesic
DIGITEK (digoxin): inotrope, antiarrhythmic, Rx: CHF, atrial fibrillation
Digoxin (LANOXIN): cardiac glycoside, Rx: CHF, dysrhythmias
Dihydrocodeine (SYNALGOS-DC): narcotic analgesic
DILANTIN (phenytoin): an anticonvulsant
DILATRATE SR (isosorbide): long-acting nitrate, Rx: angina
DILAUDID (hydromorphone): narcotic analgesic
Diltiazem (CARDIZEM): calcium blocker, Rx: angina, HTN, PSVT

Dimenhydrinate (DRAMAMINE): antihistamine, Rx: allergies
DIOCTYL (docusate): stool softener, Rx: constipation
DIOVAN (valsartan): angiotensin II inhibitor, Rx: HTN
DIOVAN HCT (valsartan, hydrochlorothiazide): angiotensin II inhibitor, diuretic, Rx: HTN
DIPENTUM (olsalazine): anti-inflammatory agent, Rx: ulcerative colitis
Diphenhydramine (BENADRYL): an antihistamine
Diphenoxylate (LOMOTIL): narcotic, Rx: diarrhea
Diphenoxylate & Atropine (LOMOTIL): narcotic, antispasmodic, Rx: diarrhea
Diphenylhydantoin (DILANTIN): anticonvulsant, Rx: seizures
DIPROLENE (betamethasone): steroid anti-inflammatory, Rx: dermatoses
DIPROLENE AF (betamethasone): steroid anti-inflammatory, Rx: dermatoses
Dipyridamole (PERSANTINE): vasodilator, Rx: angina
Dirithromycin (DYNABAC): an antibiotic
Disopyramide (NORPACE): antiarrhythmic, Rx: PVCs
Disulfiram (ANTABUSE): inhibits metabolism of alcohol, Rx: alcohol addiction
DITROPAN XL (oxybutynin): anticholinergic / antispasmodic, Rx: urinary frequency, incontinence, dysuria
DIURIL (chlorothiazide): antihypertensive / diuretic
Divalproex (DEPAKOTE): antiepileptic, Rx: seizures
Docusate (DIALOSE): stool softener
Dolasetron (ANZEMET): antiemetic, Rx: nausea and vomiting
DOLOBID (diflunisal): NSAID analgesic
DOLOPHINE (methadone): narcotic analgesic
Donepezil (ARICEPT): cholinergic, Rx: Alzheimer's disease
DONNATAL (phenobarbital, belladonna alkaloids): barbiturate sedative, antispasmodic, Rx: ulcers
Dornase Alfa (PULMOZYME): lytic enzyme that dissolves infected lung secretions, Rx: cystic fibrosis
DORYX (doxycycline): an antibiotic
Dorzolamide (TRUSOPT): Rx: glaucoma, reduces IOP
DOVONEX (calcipotriene): vitamin D, Rx: psoriasis
Doxazosin (CARDURA): alpha blocker, Rx: HTN, prostatic hypertrophy
Doxepin (SINEQUAN): tricyclic antidepressant
DOXIL (doxorubicin): antineoplastic, Rx: AIDS-related tumors
Doxorubicin (DOXIL): antineoplastic, Rx: AIDS-related tumors
Doxycycline (VIBRAMYCIN): an antibiotic
Doxylamine (UNISOM): antihistamine sedative, Rx: insomnia
DRAMAMINE (dimenhydrinate): an antinauseant

Dronabinol (MARINOL): appetite stimulant, Rx: weight loss in chemotherapy, cancer, AIDS
DTIC-DOME (dacarbazine): anticancer agent, Rx: melanomas, Hodgkin's disease
DUONEB (ipratropium, albuterol): bronchodilators, Rx: asthma, COPD
DURAGESIC (fentanyl): transdermal narcotic analgesic
DURAMORPH (morphine): a narcotic analgesic
DURATUSS AM/PM PACK GP (guaifenesin, pseudoephedrine): decongestant, expectorant, Rx: colds
DYAZIDE (HCTZ, triamterene): antihypertensive / diuretic, Rx: HTN
DYNABAC (dirithromycin): an antibiotic
DYNACIN (minocycline): an antibiotic
DYNACIRC CR (isradipine): calcium blocker, Rx: HTN, angina
DYRENIUM (triamterene): potassium-sparing diuretic, Rx: CHF

E

EC-NAPROSYN (naproxen): NSAID analgesic, Rx: arthritis, pain, inflammation, H/A
EDECRIN (ethacrynic acid): a diuretic, Rx: CHF
EES (erythromycin): an antibiotic
Efavirenz (SUSTIVA): antiviral, Rx: HIV-I infection
EFFEXOR, EFFEXOR XR (venlafaxine): antidepressant
ELDEPRYL (selegiline): MAO inhibitor, Rx: Parkinson's disease
ELIMITE (permethrin): topical scabicidal agent, Rx: scabies, lice
ELMIRON (pentosan): urinary tract analgesic, Rx: cystitis
ELOCON (mometasone): topical steroid anti-inflammatory
Eloxatin (oxaliplatin): antineoplastic, Rx: colorectal cancer
ELSPAR (asparginase): antineoplastic, Rx: leukemia, sarcoma
EMCYT (estramustine): anticancer agent, Rx: prostate CA
EMGEL (erythromycin): an antibiotic, Rx: infection
EMTRIVA (emtricitabine): antiviral, Rx: HIV / AIDS
ENABLEX (darifenacin): antispasmodic, Rx: urinary incontinence
Enalapril, Enalaprilat (VASOTEC): ACE inhibitor, Rx: HTN, CHF
ENDOCET (oxycodone, acetaminophen): narcotic analgesic
ENDODAN (hydrocodone, acetaminophen): narcotic analgesic
ENDURON (methyclothiazide): antihypertensive / diuretic, Rx: HTN
ENJUVIA (plant-derived estrogen): hormone, Rx: menopause symptoms

ENLON-PLUS (edrophonium, atropine): anticholinesterase, Rx: myasthenia gravis

ENPRESSE (levonorgestrel, ethinyl estradiol): oral contraceptive

Entacapone (COMTAN): COMT inhibitor, Rx: Parkinson's disease

ENTOCORT EC (budesonide): steroid anti-inflammatory, Rx: Crohn's disease

Ephedrine (RYNATUSS): a bronchodilator, Rx: asthma, COPD

EPIFOAM (hydrocortisone, pramoxine): anti-inflammatory, antipruritic, local anesthetic, Rx: dermatosis

EPIPEN (epinephrine): bronchodilator / vasoconstrictor, Rx: allergic reaction

EPIVIR, EPIVIR HBV (lamivudine): antiviral, Rx: HIV, Hepatitis B

Epoetin Alfa (EPOGEN): increases RBC production, Rx: anemia

EPOGEN (epoetin alfa): increases RBC production, Rx: anemia

EQUETRO (carbamazepine): anticonvulsant, Rx: bipolar disorder, seizures, neuralgia

ERBITUX (cetuximab): anticancer agent, Rx: colorectal cancer

ERGAMISOL (levamisole): immunomodulator, Rx: colon CA

Ergocalciferol (CALCIFEROL): vitamin D, Rx: hypocalcemia, hypoparathyroidism, rickets, osteodystrophy

ERRIN (norethindrone): oral contraceptive

ERYC DELAYED RELEASE (erythromycin): an antibiotic

ERYGEL (erythromycin): antibiotic, Rx: infection, acne

ERYPED 200, 400 (erythromycin): antibiotic, Rx: infection

ERY-TAB (erythromycin): an antibiotic

Erythromycin (EES): an antibiotic

ESGIC (APAP, caffeine, butalbital): analgesic / muscle relaxant / antianxiety compound, Rx: headache

ESGIC-PLUS (butalbital, APAP, caffeine): sedative / analgesic

ESKALITH, ESKALITH CR (lithium): a tranquilizer, Rx: mania, depression

Esomeprazole (NEXIUM): suppresses gastric acid pump, Rx: esophagitis, GERD, gastric ulcers

Estazolam (PROSOM): sedative / hypnotic, Rx: insomnia

ESTRACE (estradiol): estrogen, Rx: menopause

ESTRADERM (estradiol): topical estrogen, Rx: menopause

Estradiol (CLIMARA): estrogen, Rx: menopause

Estramustine (EMCYT): antineoplastic, Rx: prostate cancer

ESTRATEST, ESTRATEST HS (estrogens, methyltestosterone): Rx: menopause

ESTRING (estrogen): hormone, Rx: urogenital symptoms, postmenopause
Estrogens (ESTRATEST): hormone, Rx: menopause
Estropipate (ORTHO-EST): estrogens, Rx: menopause
ESTROSTEP FE, 21 (norethindrone, estradiol, iron): oral contraceptive, Rx: pregnancy prophylaxis
Ethacrynate (EDECRIN): diuretic, Rx: pulmonary edema
Ethinyl Estradiol (ORTHO-NOVUM): oral contraceptive
Ethionamide (TRECATOR SC): antibiotic, Rx: tuberculosis
Ethosuximide (ZARONTIN): anticonvulsant, Rx: absence Sz
Etidronate (DIDRONEL): bone metabolism regulator, Rx:
Etodolac (LODINE): NSAID analgesic, Rx: arthritis
Etoposide (VEPESID): antineoplastic, Rx: testicular cancer, lung cancer
EULEXIN (flutamide): antiandrogenic, anticancer agent, Rx: prostate cancer
EVISTA (raloxifene): Rx: osteoporosis prevention
EVOXAC (cevimeline): cholinergic, Rx: dry mouth from Sjogren's syndrome
EXELON (rivastigmine): cholinesterase inhibitor, Rx: Alzheimer's disease
EXTENDRYL (phenylephrine, methscopolamine, chlorpheniramine): antihistamine, decongestant, Rx: allergies
EXTENDRYL SYRUP (phenylephrine, methscopolamine, chlorpheniramine): decongestant, antihistamine, Rx: allergies
EXUBERA (inhaled insulin): hypoglycemic, Rx: diabetes

F

FACTIVE (gemifloxacin): an antibiotic
Famciclovir (FAMVIR): antiviral, Rx: herpes
Famotidine (PEPCID): H-2 blocker, inhibits gastric acid, Rx: ulcers
FAMVIR (famciclovir): antiviral, Rx: herpes zoster, genital herpes
FARESTON (toremifene): antiestrogen, Rx: breast cancer, post-menopause
FAZACLO (clozapine): antipsychotic, Rx: schizophrenia
Felbamate (FELBATOL): antiepileptic, Rx: seizures
FELBATOL (felbamate): antiepileptic, Rx: seizures
FELDENE (piroxicam): a NSAID analgesic
Felodipine (PLENDIL): calcium blocker, Rx: HTN, angina
FEMARA (letrozole): estrogen inhibitor, Rx: breast cancer
FEMHRT (norethindrone, estradiol): hormones, Rx: osteoporosis prevention, menopause

Fenofibrate (TRICOR): lipid regulator, Rx: hyperlipidemia

Fenoprofen (NALFON): NSAID analgesic

Fentanyl (DURAGESIC): narcotic analgesic, Rx: pain relief

FERRLECIT (sodium ferric gluconate): hematinic,
Rx: irondeficiency anemia, hemodialysis

Fexofenadine (ALLEGRA): antihistamine, Rx: allergies

Filgrastim (NEUPOGEN): white blood cell stimulator,
Rx: cancer, chemotherapy, bone marrow transplant

Finasteride (PROPECIA): dihydrotestosterone inhibitor,
Rx: hair loss, baldness, BPH

FLAGYL (metronidazole): an antimicrobial agent

Flecainide (TAMBOCOR): antiarrhythmic, Rx: PSVT,
paroxysmal atrial fibrillation, VT

FLEXERIL (cyclobenzaprine): skeletal muscle relaxant

FLOLAN (epoprostenol): vasodilator, platelet inhibitor
Rx: pulmonary hypertension

FLOMAX (tamsulosin): alpha-1 blocker, Rx: enlarged prostate

FLONASE (fluticasone): steroid, Rx: allergic rhinitis

FLOVENT (fluticasone): steroid anti-inflammatory, Rx: asthma

FLOXIN (ofloxacin): an antibiotic

Floxuridine (FUDR): antineoplastic, Rx: liver, GI cancer

Fluconazole (DIFLUCAN): an antifungal agent

Flucytosine (ANCOBON): antifungal, Rx: candida,
cryptococcus infection

FLUDARA (fludarabine): antiviral, antimetabolite
Rx: lymphocytic leukemia

Fludarabine (FLUDARA): antiviral, antimetabolite
Rx: lymphocytic leukemia

FLUMADINE (rimantadine): antiviral, Rx: influenza A

Flunisolide (AEROBID): steroid anti-inflammatory, Rx: asthma

Fluocinolone (CAPEX): steroid anti-inflammatory,
Rx: dermatoses

Fluocinonide (LIDEX): steroid anti-inflammatory,
Rx: dermatoses, pruritus

Fluorouracil (EFUDEX): anticancer agent, Rx: solar keratosis
carcinomas

Fluoxetine (PROZAC): antidepressant, Rx: depression,
obsessive-compulsive disorder

Fluphenazine: antipsychotic, Rx: schizophrenia, delusions,
hallucinations

Flurazepam (DALMANE): sedative-hypnotic, Rx: insomnia

Flurbiprofen: NSAID analgesic, Rx: arthritis

Flutamide (EULEXIN): antiandrogenic, anticancer agent,
Rx: prostate cancer

Fluvastatin (LESCOL): cholesterol reducer

Fluvoxamine (LUVOX): antidepressant, Rx: depression
FOCALIN (dexmethylphenidate): stimulant, Rx: ADHD
Folic Acid (VITAFOL-OB): vitamin coenzyme, Rx: anemia
FORTAMET (metformin): oral hypoglycemic, Rx: diabetes
FORTAZ (ceftazidime): an antibiotic
FORTOVASE (saquinavir): antiviral, Rx: HIV
FOSAMAX (alendronate): reduces bone loss, Rx: osteoporosis, Paget's disease
Foscarnet (FOSCAVIR): antiviral, Rx: herpes
FOSCAVIR (foscarnet): antiviral, Rx: herpes
Fosfomycin (NONUROL): antibacterial, Rx: UTI
FOSFREE (calcium, iron): minerals, Rx: dietary supplement
Fosinopril (MONOPRIL): ACE inhibitor, Rx: HTN
Fosphenytoin (CEREBYX): anticonvulsant, Rx: seizures
FROVA (frovatriptan): antimigraine, Rx: migraine headaches
FUNGOID (clotrimazole): antifungal, Rx: fungal infection
Furosemide (LASIX): diuretic, Rx: CHF, hypertension
FUZEON (enfuvirtide): antiviral, fusion inhibitor, Rx: HIV / AIDS

G

Gabapentin (NEURONTIN): antiepileptic / analgesic, Rx: seizures, postherpetic neuralgia, herpes zoster, shingles
GABITRIL (tiagabine): antiepileptic, Rx: partial seizures
Ganciclovir (CYTOVENE): antiviral, Rx: CMV in AIDS, and other immunocompromised pts
GASTROCROM (cromolyn): antiasthmatic, antiallergic, Rx: diarrhea, H/A, urticaria, PSS
Gemfibrozil (LOPID): lowers serum lipids
GEMZAR (gemcitabine): antineoplastic, Rx: lung, pancreatic CA
GENGRAF (cyclosporine): immunosuppressive, Rx: rheumatoid arthritis, psoriasis, prevention of kidney, heart, liver transplant rejection
GENOTROPIN (somatropin): growth stimulator, Rx: AIDS, wasting syndrome, growth disorders
Gentamicin (GARAMYCIN): an antibiotic
GEOCILLIN (carbenicillin): an antibiotic
GEODON (ziprasidone): antipsychotic, Rx: schizophrenia
Glatiramir (COPAXONE): modifies immune response, Rx: MS
GLEEVEC (imatinib): anticancer agent, Rx: leukemia, gastrointestinal cancer
GLIADEL WAFER (polifeprosan): oncolytic agent, Rx: malignant glioma
Glimepiride (AMARYL): oral hypoglycemic, Rx: diabetes

Glipizide (GLUCOTROL): oral hypoglycemic, Rx: diabetes
Glucagon: hormone, mobilizes glucose, Rx: hypoglycemia
GLUCOPHAGE (metformin): oral hypoglycemic, Rx: diabetes
Glucosamine (COSAMIN-DS): cartilage growth stimulator
GLUCOTROL (glipizide): oral hypoglycemic, Rx: diabetes
GLUCOVANCE (glyburide, metformin): oral hypoglycemic
GLUMETZA (metformin): oral hypoglycemic, Rx: diabetes
Glyburide (DIABETA): oral hypoglycemic, Rx: diabetes
Glycopyrrolate (ROBINUL): anticholinergic, Rx: peptic ulcers
GLYNASE (glyburide): oral hypoglycemic, Rx: diabetes
GLYSET (miglitol): oral hypoglycemic, Rx: diabetes
GORDOCHOM (chloroxylenol): antifungal, Rx: ringworm, athlete's foot
Goserelin (ZOLADEX): antineoplastic, Rx: prostate CA, endometriosis
Granisetron (KYTRIL): antiemetic, Rx: chemotherapy, nausea
GRIFULVIN V (griseofulvin): antifungal, Rx: ringworm
Griseofulvin (FULVICIN): antifungal, Rx: ringworm
Gris-PEG (griseofulvin): antifungal, Rx: ringworm
Guanfacine (TENEX): antihypertensive, Rx: HTN
GYNAZOLE-I (butoconazole): antifungal, Rx: yeast infections
GYNODIOL (estradiol): hormone, Rx: vaginitis, menopause, breast cancer, osteoporosis

H

HALCION (triazolam): a benzodiazepine hypnotic, Rx: insomnia
HALDOL (haloperidol): a major tranquilizer
Halobetasol (ULTRAVATE): steroid anti-inflammatory, Rx: pruritus
Haloperidol (HALDOL): antipsychotic, Rx: psychosis, hyperactivity
HCT, HCTZ (hydrochlorothiazide): antihypertensive / diuretic
HEMOCYTE (iron): iron supplement
Hesperidin (PERIDIN-C): antioxidant, Rx: dietary supplement
HEXALEN (altretamine): anticancer agent, Rx: ovarian cancer
HIVID (zalcitabine) antiviral, Rx: AIDS
HUMALOG (insulin): hypoglycemic, Rx: diabetes mellitus
HUMATROPE (somatropin): human growth hormone
HUMIRA (adalimumab): immune system inhibitor, Rx: rheumatoid and psoriatic arthritis, and ankylosing spondylitis
HUMULIN N, HUMULIN R (insulin): hypoglycemic, Rx: diabetes

HYCAMTIN (topotecan): antineoplastic, Rx: ovarian, hepatic CA

HYCODAN (hydrocodone, homatropine): narcotic antitussive

HYCOMINE COMPOUND (hydrocodone, chlorpheniramine, APAP, caffeine, phenylephrine): narcotic antitussive / antihistamine / decongestant, Rx: colds, URI

HYCOTUSS (hydrocodone, guaifenesin): narcotic antitussive / expectorant

Hydralazine (APRESOLINE): antihypertensive agent

HYDRA-ZIDE (hydralazine, HCTZ): antihypertensive / diuretic

Hydrochlorothiazide (HCTZ): antihypertensive / diuretic

Hydrocodone: narcotic analgesic / antitussive

Hydrocodone with APAP: narcotic analgesic compound

Hydrocortisone (CORTEF): steroid anti-inflammatory agent

HYDROCORTONE (hydrocortisone): steroid anti-inflammatory

HYDRODIURIL (HCTZ): antihypertensive / diuretic

Hydromorphone (DILAUDID): narcotic analgesic / antitussive

Hydroquinone (MELANEX): Rx: pigmentation disorders

Hydroxychloroquine (PLAQUENIL): antimalarial, Rx: malaria, lupus, arthritis

Hydroxypropyl (LACRISERT): opthalmic lubricant, Rx: dry eyes

Hydroxyurea anticancer agent, elastogenic, Rx: melanoma, leukemia, ovarian CA, sickle cell anemia

Hydroxyzine (ATARAX): sedative / tranquilizer / antihistamine

Hylan (SYNVISC): intraarticular elastoviscous polymer fluid, Rx: osteoarthritis

Hyoscyamine (CYSTOSPAS): an antispasmodic, Rx: lower urinary tract and GI tract spasm

HYTRIN (terazosin): an antihypertensive agent

HYZAAR (losartan, HCTZ): antihypertensive compound

I

IBERET (iron, vitamins, mineral): vitamin / mineral supplement

Ibutilide (CORVERT): antiarrhythmic, Rx: Atrial Fib, Atrial Flutter

ILETIN (insulin preparations): Rx: diabetes mellitus

Imatinib (GLEEVEC): anticancer agent, Rx: leukemia, GI cancer

Imipenem (PRIMAXIN): antibiotic, Rx: infections

Imipramine (TOFRANIL): a tricyclic antidepressant

Imiquimod (ALDARA): immune system modifier, Rx: genital warts

IMITREX (sumatriptan): Rx: migraine H/A

IMODIUM (loperamide): slows peristalsis, Rx: diarrhea
IMODIUM A-D (loperamide): anti-diarrhea agent
IMURAN (azathioprine): immunosuppressant, Rx: organ transplants, ulcerative colitis, lupus, severe arthritis
Indapamide (LOZOL): an antihypertensive / diuretic
INDERAL, INDERAL LA (propranolol): beta blocker, Rx: HTN, angina, cardiac dysrhythmias, AMI, and migraine H/A
INDOCIN, INDOCIN SR (indomethacin): NSAID , Rx: arthritis
Indomethacin (INDOCIN): NSAID analgesic, Rx: arthritis
INFERGEN (interferon alfacon-1): antiviral, Rx: hepatitis C
Infliximab (REMICADE): neutralizes tumor necrosis factor, Rx: Crohn's disease
INH (isoniazid): antibiotic, Rx: tuberculosis
INSPRA (eplerenone): aldosterone blocker, Rx: HTN, CHF
Insulin (HUMULIN): hypoglycemic, Rx: diabetes mellitus
INTAL (cromolyn): anti-inflammatory, Rx: asthma
INVEGA (paliperidone): antipsychotic, Rx: schizophrenia
INVERSINE (mecamylamine): an antihypertensive agent
INVIRASE (saquinavir): protease inhibitor antiviral, Rx: HIV/AIDS
IONAMIN (phentermine): stimulant, Rx: appetite suppression
Ipratropium (ATROVENT): bronchodilator
Irbesartan (AVAPRO): antihypertensive, Rx: hypertension
Isoniazid (RIFAMATE): antibiotic, Rx: tuberculosis
Isoproterenol: ß-bronchodilator, Rx: asthma, COPD
ISOPTIN SR (verapamil): calcium blocker, Rx: angina, HTN, PSVT prophylaxis, headache
Isosorbide dinitrate (ISORDIL): long-acting nitrate, Rx: angina
Isosorbide mononitrate: long-acting nitrate, Rx: angina

J

JANUVIA (sitagliptin): oral hypoglycemic, Rx: diabetes
JOLIVETTE (norethindrone): oral contraceptive
JUNEL, FE (norethindrone, estradiol): oral contraceptive

K

KADIAN (morphine): narcotic analgesic
KALETRA (lopinavir, ritonavir): antivirals, Rx: HIV, AIDS
Kaolin-Pectin (KAOPECTATE): stool binder, Rx: diarrhea
KAOPECTATE (kaolin, pectin): stool binder, Rx: diarrhea
KARIVA (desogrestel, ethinyl estradiol): oral contraceptive
K-DUR (KCl): a potassium supplement
KEFLEX (cephalexin): an antibiotic
KEPPRA (levatiracetam): antiepileptic, Rx: seizures

KERLONE (betaxolol): beta-1 blocker, Rx: HTN
Ketoconazole (NIZORAL): an antifungal agent
Ketoprofen (ORUDIS): NSAID, Rx: arthritis
Ketorolac (TORADOL): NSAID analgesic
Ketotifen (ZADITOR): antihistamine, anti-inflammatory,
Rx: allergic conjunctivitis
Kineret (anakinra) DMARD / interleukin-1 blocker,
Rx: rheumatoid arthritis
KLARON (sulfacetamide): an antibacterial
KLONOPIN (clonazepam): a benzodiazepine hypnotic, Rx: Sz
KLOR-CON (KCl): a potassium supplement
KOGENATE (antihemophilic Factor VIII), Rx: hemophilia
K-PHOS (potassium phosphate): potassium ion
KRISTALOSE (lactulose): stool softener, Rx: constipation
KRONOFED-A (pseudoephedrine, chlorpheniramine):
decongestant, antihistamine, Rx: colds, allergies
K-TAB (KCl): potassium supplement
KUTRASE (digestive enzymes, hyoscyamine,
phenyltoloxamine): antispasmodic / sedative, Rx: indigestion
KU-ZYME (digestive enzymes): Rx: indigestion
KWELL (lindane): parasiticide, Rx: lice, scabies
KYTRIL (granisetron): antinauseant / antiemetic

L

Labetalol (NORMODYNE): beta blocker, Rx: HTN, angina
Lactulose (KRISTALOSE): laxative, Rx: constipation
LAMICTAL (lamotrigine): anticonvulsant, Rx: seizures
LAMISIL (terbinafine): antifungal, Rx: fungal infections
Lamivudine (EPIVIR): antiviral, Rx: HIV
Lamotrigine (LAMICTAL): anticonvulsant, Rx: seizures, bipolar
disorder
LANOXICAPS (digoxin): cardiac glycoside, Rx: CHF,
dysrhythmias
LANOXIN (digoxin): cardiac glycoside, Rx: CHF, dysrhythmias
Lansoprazole (PREVACID): suppresses gastic acid, Rx: ulcers
LANTUS (insulin): hypoglycemic agent, Rx: diabetes
LARIAM (mefloquine): antimalarial agent
LASIX (furosemide): diuretic, Rx: HTN, CHF
Leflunomide (ARAVA): antiarthritic, anti-inflammatory,
Rx: rheumatoid arthritis
LESCOL (fluvastatin): cholesterol reducer
LESSINA (levonorgestrel, ethinyl estradiol): oral contraceptive
LEUKERAN (chlorambucil): anticancer agent, Rx: leukemia,
lymphoma, Hodgkin's disease

Leuprolide (LUPRON): hormone, Rx: endometriosis
Levalbuterol (XOPENEX): ß-2 bronchodilator, Rx: COPD, asthma
Levamisole (ERGAMISOLE): immunostimulant, Rx: colon CA
LEVAQUIN (levofloxacin): antibacterial, Rx: pneumonia
Levatiracetam (KEPPRA): antiepileptic, Rx: seizures
LEVATOL (penbutolol): beta blocker, Rx: hypertension
LEVBID (hyoscyamine): antispasmodic, Rx: ulcers
LEVEMIR (insulin): hypoglycemic, Rx: diabetes
LEVITRA (vardenafil): vasodilator, Rx: male erectile dysfunction
LEVLEN 21, 28 (levonorgestrel, estradiol): oral contraceptive
Levodopa (SINEMET): dopamine precursor, Rx: Parkinson's disease
Levofloxacin (LEVAQUIN): antibacterial, Rx: pneumonia
Levonorgestrel (NORPLANT): implanted contraceptive
LEVORA (levonorgestrel, estradiol): oral contraceptive
Levorphanol (LEVO-DROMORAN): a narcotic analgesic
LEVOTHROID (levothyroxine): thyroid hormone
Levothyroxine (SYNTHROID): thyroid hormone
LEVOXYL (levothyroxine): thyroid hormone
LEVSIN, LEVSINEX (hyoscyamine): antispasmodic, Rx: ulcers
LEXAPRO (escitalopram): SSRI antidepressant, Rx: depression
LEXXEL (enalapril, felodipine): ACE inhibitor, calcium blocker, Rx: HTN
LIBRIUM (chlordiazepoxide): anxiolytic / sedative, Rx: anxiety
LIDEX (fluocinonide): steroid anti-inflammatory, Rx: pruritus
LINCOCIN (lincomycin): an antibiotic
Lindane (KWELL): parasiticide, Rx: scabies
Liothyronine (CYTOMEL): thyroid hormone
Liotrix (THYROLAR): thyroid hormone
LIPITOR (atorvastatin): antihyperlipidemic, Rx: high cholesterol
Lisinopril (ZESTRIL): ACE inhibitor, Rx: HTN, CHF, AMI
Lisinopril, HCTZ (ZESTORETIC): ACE inhibitor, Rx: HTN, CHF, AMI
Lithium (LITHOBID): antimanic, Rx: depression, mania
LITHOBID (lithium): antimanic agent, Rx: depression, mania
LO/OVRAL, LO/OVRAL 28: an oral contraceptive
LOCOID (hydrocortisone): steroid anti-inflammatory
LODRANE 12D Capsules (brompheniramine, pseudoephedrine): antihistamine / decongestant
LODRANE Liquid (brompheniramine, pseudoephedrine): antihistamine / decongestant
LODRANE Tablets (brompheniramine): antihistamine
LOESTRIN 21, FE (norethindrone, estradiol): oral contraceptive

150

Drugs

151

LOMOTIL (diphenoxylate, atropine): narcotic antidiarrheal / antispasmodic compound
LONITEN (minoxidil): vasodilator / antihypertensive
LONOX (diphenoxylate, atropine): narcotic antidiarrheal / antispasmodic compound
Loperamide (IMODIUM): antidiarrheal agent
LOPID (gemfibrozil): lowers serum lipids
Lopinavir (KALETRA): antiviral, Rx: HIV, AIDS
LOPRESSOR (metoprolol): beta-1 blocker, Rx: hypertension
LOPRESSOR HCT (metoprolol, hydrochlorothiazide): beta-1 blocker, diuretic, Rx: hypertension
LOPROX (ciclopirox): antifungal, Rx: ringworm, candida
LORABID (loracarbef): antibiotic, Rx: sinusitis
Lorazepam (ATIVAN): a benzodiazepine hypnotic
LORCET 10/650, LORCET HD, LORCET PLUS (hydrocodone, APAP): narcotic analgesic compound
LORTAB (hydrocodone, APAP): narcotic analgesic
Losartan (COZAAR): antihypertensive, Rx: HTN
LOTENSIN (benazepril): ACE inhibitor, Rx: HTN, CHF
LOTREL (amlodipine, benazepril): calcium blocker / ACE inhibitor, Rx: HTN
LOTRIMIN (clotrimazole): an antifungal agent
LOTRISONE (clotrimazole, betamethasone): topical antifungal / steroid anti-inflammatory compound
LOTRONEX (alosetron): antidiarrheal, Rx: irritable bowel synd.
Lovastatin (MEVACOR): lowers serum cholesterol
LOW-OGESTREL 28 (norgestrel, estradiol): oral contraceptive
Loxapine (LOXITANE): an antipsychotic, Rx: schizophrenia
LOXITANE (loxapine): a tranquilizer
LUCENTIS (ranibizumab): blood vessel growth inhibitor, Rx: macular degeneration
LUMIGAN (bimatoprost): lowers intraocular pressure, Rx: glaucoma
LUPRON DEPOT (leuprolide): hormone, Rx: endometriosis
LUVOX (fluvoxamine): SSRI antidepressant, Rx: schizophrenia, obsessive compulsive disorder
LYRICA (pregabalin): anticonvulsant, Rx: partial seizures, neuropathic pain

M

MACROBID (nitrofurantoin): antibacterial, Rx: UTI
MACRODANTIN (nitrofurantoin): antibacterial, Rx: UTI
MALARONE (atovaquone, proguanil): antimalarial agents

Malathion (OVIDE): organophosphate insecticide, Rx: head lice

Maprotiline (LUDIOMIL): cyclic antidepressant

MARINOL (dronabinol): appetite stimulant, Rx: weight loss in AIDS, chemotherapy

MAVIK (trandolapril): ACE inhibitor, Rx: HTN

MAXAIR (pirbuterol): beta-2 stimulant, Rx: asthma, COPD

MAXALT (rizatriptan): antimigraine, Rx: migraine headaches

MAXIDEX (dexamethasone): steroid anti-inflammatory eye drops

MAXIDONE (hydrocodone, APAP): narcotic analgesic compound

MAXZIDE (triamterene, HCTZ): antihypertensive / diuretic, Rx: HTN

MEBARAL (mephobarbital): barbiturate sedative, Rx: epilepsy, anxiety

Meclizine (ANTIVERT): antinauseant, Rx: vertigo

Meclofenamate: NSAID, Rx: arthritis, pain, dysmenorrhea, heavy menstrual blood loss

Medroxyprogesterone: hormone, Rx: endometriosis, amenorrhea, uterine bleeding, contraception

MEFOXIN (cefoxitin): an antibiotic

Megestrol (MEGACE): appetite stimulant, Rx: anorexia with AIDS; also an antineoplastic, Rx: breast, endometrial CA

MENEST (estrogens): hormones, Rx: menopause, breast CA, prostatic CA

MENOSTAR (estradiol): transdermal hormone, Rx: osteoporosis

MENTAX (butenafine): antifungal, Rx: ringworm, athlete's foot

Meperidine (DEMEROL): narcotic analgesic

MEPHYTON (vitamin K-1): Rx: coagulation disorders

Meprobamate (MILTOWN): a tranquilizer

MEPRON (atovaquone) antibiotic, Rx: pneumocystis carinii pneumonia in AIDS

MERIDIA (sibutramine): stimulant, Rx: obesity

MESTINON (pyridostigmine): anticholinesterase, Rx: myasthenia gravis

METADATE CD, ER (methylphenidate): stimulant, Rx: ADHD

METAGLIP (glipizide, metformin): hypoglycemics, Rx: diabetes

Metaproterenol (ALUPENT): ß-2 bronchodilator, Rx: COPD, asthma

Metformin (GLUCOPHAGE): oral hypoglycemic, Rx: diabetes

Methadone (DOLOPHINE): narcotic analgesic

METHADOSE (methadone): narcotic analgesic

Methamphetamine (DESOXYN): stimulant appetite suppressant, Rx: ADD, obesity
Methazolamide: reduces intraocular pressure, Rx: glaucoma
Methenamine (URISED): antiseptic, Rx: UTI, cystitis
Methimazole (TAPAZOLE): Rx: antithyroid, Rx: hyperthyroidism
Methocarbamol (ROBAXIN): skeletal muscle antispasmodic
Methotrexate: anticancer agent, Rx: psoriasis, arthritis
Methscopolamine (PAMINE): anticholinergic, Rx: peptic ulcer
Methsuximide (CELONTIN): anticonvulsant, Rx: absence Sz
Methyclothiazide (AQUATENSEN): antihypertensive / diuretic
Methyldopa (ALDOMET): an antihypertensive
Methylphenidate (RITALIN): stimulant, Rx: ADHD, narcolepsy
Methylprednisolone (MEDROL): steroid anti-inflammatory
Metoclopramide (REGLAN): improves gastric emptying, Rx: heartburn, ulcers
Metolazone (ZAROXOLYN): antihypertensive / diuretic
Metoprolol (TOPROL-XL): cardioselective ß-blocker, Rx: HTN, angina, arrhythmias
Metronidazole (FLAGYL): an antimicrobial agent
MEVACOR (lovastatin): lowers serum cholesterol
Mexiletine (MEXITIL): an antiarrhythmic
MEXITIL (mexiletine): an antiarrhythmic
MIACALCIN (calcitonin-salmon): bone resorption inhibitor hormone, Rx: hypercalcemia, Paget's disease, osteoporosis
MICARDIS (telmisartan): ACE inhibitor, Rx: HTN
Miconazole (MONISTAT): antifungal, Rx: candidiasis
MICRONASE (glyburide): oral hypoglycemic, Rx: diabetes
MICROZIDE (HCTZ): thiazide antihypertensive / diuretic
MIDAMOR (amiloride): a potassium-sparing diuretic
Midazolam: sedative / anxiolytic
Midodrine (PROAMATINE): vasopressor, Rx: orthostatic hypotension
MIDRIN (isometheptene, dichloralphenazone, APAP): vasoconstrictor / sedative / analgesic, Rx: H/A
Miglitol (GLYCET): oral hypoglycemic, Rx: diabetes
MINIPRESS (prazosin): alpha-1 blocker, Rx: hypertension
MINITRAN (transdermal nitroglycerin): nitrate, Rx: angina
MINIZIDE (prazosin, polythiazide): an antihypertensive
MINOCIN (minocycline): an antibiotic
Minocycline (MINOCIN): an antibiotic
MIRALAX (polyethylene glycol): a laxative
MIRAPEX (pramipexole): dopamine agonist, Rx: Parkinson's disease
Mirtazapine (REMERON): antidepressant, Rx: depression

Misoprostol (CYTOTEC): antiulcer, Rx: prevents gastric ulcers caused by NSAIDS
MOBAN (molindone): a tranquilizer
MOBIC (meloxicam): NSAID analgesic
Modafinil (PROVIGIL): wakefulness-promoting agent, Rx: narcolepsy, daytime sleepiness
MODURETIC (amiloride, HCTZ): antihypertensive / diuretic
Moexipril (UNIVASC): ACE inhibitor, Rx: HTN
Mometasone (ELOCON): topical steroid anti-inflammatory
MONOCAL (fluoride, calcium): mineral supplement
MONODOX (doxycycline): an antibiotic
MONOKET (isosorbide mononitrate): nitrate, Rx: angina
MONOPRIL (fosinopril): ACE inhibitor, Rx: HTN
MONUROL (fosfomycin): antibiotic, Rx: UTI
Morphine sulfate: a narcotic analgesic
MOTOFEN (difenoxin, atropine): narcotic antidiarrheal agent
Moxifloxacin (AVELOX): antibiotic, Rx: bronchitis, pneumonia
MS CONTIN (morphine): a narcotic analgesic
MSIR Capsules, Solution, Concentrate (morphine): a narcotic analgesic
MYCOBUTIN (rifabutin): antibiotic, Rx: AIDS
Mycophenolate (CELLCEPT): immunosuppressant, Rx: organ transplants
MYKROX (metolazone): an antihypertensive / diuretic
MYLERAN (busulfan): anticancer agent, Rx: leukemia

N

Nabumetone (RELAFEN): NSAID, Rx: arthritis
Nadolol (CORGARD): ß-blocker, Rx: HTN, angina, arrhythmias
Nafarelin (SYNAREL): hormone, Rx: endometriosis, precocious puberty, decreased gonadal steroids
Naftifine (NAFTIN): antifungal, Rx: fungal infections
NAFTIN (naftifine): topical antifungal agent
Nalbuphine (NUBAINE): narcotic analgesic, Rx: pain relief
Nalmefene (REVEX): narcotic antidote, Rx: narcotic overdose
Naltrexone (REVIA): opioid antagonist; alcohol deterrent
NAMENDA (memantine): NMDA antagonist, Rx: Alzheimer's disease
Nandrolone (DECA-DURABOLIN): anabolic steroid, androgenizing hormone, Rx: anemia, breast cancer
Naphazoline (NAPHCON): steroid anti-inflammatory, Rx: itching eyes, ocular congestion
NAPHCON-A (pheniramine, naphazoline): antihistamine, steroid anti-inflammatory, Rx: itching eyes, redness

Naratriptan (AMERGE): antimigraine, Rx: acute migraine H/A
NARDIL (phenelzine): MAO inhibitor, Rx: depression, bulimia
NASACORT AQ (triamcinolone): steroid anti-inflammatory, Rx: allergies
NASAREL (flunisolide): steroid anti-inflammatory, Rx: rhinitis
NASCOBAL (cyanocobalamin): vitamin B-12, Rx: anemia
NASONEX (mometasone): steroid anti-inflammatory, Rx: allergic rhinitis
NATRECOR (nesiritide): b-type natriuretic peptide vasodilator, Rx: CHF
NAVANE (thiothixene): a major tranquilizer
NECON (norethindrone, estradiol): oral contraceptive
Nedocromil (TILADE): anti-inflammatory, Rx: asthma
Nefazodone (SERZONE): antidepressant, Rx: depression
Nelfinavir (VIRACEPT): protease inhibitor antiviral, Rx: HIV
NEMBUTAL (pentobarbital): barbiturate sedative / hypnotic
NEODECADRON (neomycin, dexamethasone): antibiotic / steroid anti-inflammatory
Neomycin (NEOSPORIN): antibiotic
NEORAL (cyclosporine): immunosuppressant, Rx: organ transplant
NEPHROCAPS (vitamins): vitamin supplement, Rx: uremia, renal failure
NEPTAZANE (methazolamide): reduces aqueous humor production, Rx: glaucoma
NESACAINE (chloroprocaine): local anesthetic
NEURONTIN (gabapentin): an antiepileptic
Nevirapine (VIRAMUNE): antiviral, Rx: HIV, AIDS
NEXIUM (esomeprazole): suppresses gastric acid pump, Rx: ulcers, esophagitis
Niacin (vitamin B-3): reduces serum cholesterol
NIACOR (niacin): vitamin B-3, Rx: lowers serum cholesterol
NIASPAN (niacin): vitamin B-3, Rx: reduces serum cholesterol
Nicardipine (CARDENE): calcium blocker, Rx: angina, HTN
NICODERM CQ (nicotine): stop smoking aid, Rx: relief of nicotine withdrawal symptoms
NICOMIDE (vitamins, minerals): nutritional supplement, Rx: acne
NICORETTE (nicotine chewing gum): Rx: cigarette withdrawal
Nicotinic Acid (niacin): vitamin B-3, Rx: reduces cholesterol
NICOTROL NS, NICOTROL PATCH (nicotine): Rx: relief of nicotine withdrawal symptoms
Nifedipine (PROCARDIA): calcium blocker, Rx: angina, HTN
NIFEREX, NIFEREX-150 (iron): mineral, Rx: anemia
NILANDRON (nilutamide): antiandrogen, Rx: prostate CA

Nilutamide (NILANDRON): antiandrogen, Rx: prostate cancer
Nimodipine (NIMOTOP): calcium blocker, Rx: improves neuro deficits after subarachnoid hemorrhage
NIMOTOP (nimodipine): calcium channel blocker, improves neurological deficits after subarachnoid hemorrhage
NIRAVAM (alprazolam): anti-anxiety, Rx: anxiety
Nisoldipine (SULAR): calcium channel blocker, Rx: HTN
NITRO-DUR (nitroglycerin): long-acting nitrate, Rx: angina
Nitrofurantoin (FURADANTIN): antibacterial agent, Rx: UTI
Nitroglycerin (NITROSTAT): vasodilator, Rx: angina
NITROLINGUAL SPRAY (nitroglycerin): nitrate, Rx: angina
NITROMIST (nitroglycerin): vasodilator lingual spray, Rx: angina
NITROSTAT (nitroglycerin): vasodilator, Rx: angina
NIX (permethrin): parasiticide, Rx: head lice
Nizatidine (AXID): histamine-2 antagonist, Rx: ulcers
NIZORAL (ketoconazole): antifungal agent, Rx: yeast infections
NOLVADEX (tamoxifen): anticancer agent, Rx: breast CA
NORCO CIII (hydrocodone, APAP): narcotic analgesic comp.
NORDETTE: an oral contraceptive
NORDITROPIN (somatropin): growth hormone, Rx: growth failure
Norethindrone (NORINYL): oral contraceptive
NORFLEX (orphenadrine): non-narcotic analgesic
Norfloxacin (NOROXIN): antibiotic, Rx: urinary tract infections
NORGESIC (orphenadrine): non-narcotic analgesic
Norgestimate (ORTHO-CYCLEN 21): oral contraceptive
Norgestrel (LO/OVRAL): oral contraceptive
NORINYL: an oral contraceptive
NORITATE (metronidazole): antibacterial, antiprotozoal, Rx: inflammation of rosacea(acne)
NORMODYNE (labetalol): beta blocker, Rx: HTN, angina
NOROXIN (norfloxacin): urinary tract antibiotic
NORPACE, NORPACE CR (disopyramide): antiarrhythmic, Rx: PVCs
NORPLANT (levonorgestrel): contraceptive
NORPRAMIN (desipramine): a tricyclic antidepressant
NOR-QD (norethindrone): oral contraceptive
NORTREL (norethindrone, ethinyl estradiol): oral contraceptive
Nortriptyline (PAMELOR): a tricyclic antidepressant
NORVASC (amlodipine): calcium blocker, Rx: HTN, angina
NORVIR (ritonavir): protease inhibitor antiviral, Rx: HIV
NOVANTRONE (mitoxantrone): antineoplastic, Rx: prostate cancer, MS
NOVOLIN (insulin): hypoglycemic, Rx: diabetes mellitus

NOVOLOG (insulin): hypoglycemic hormone, Rx: diabetes
NOVOLOG MIX 70/30 (insulin): hypoglycemic, Rx: diabetes
NUBAIN (nalbuphine): a narcotic analgesic
NULEV (hyoscyamine): antispasmodic, Rx: peptic ulcers
NUMORPHAN (oxymorphone): a narcotic analgesic
Nystatin (MYCOSTATIN): an antifungal agent
NYSTOP (nystatin): antifungal, Rx: candida

O

OBEGYN: vitamins and minerals
Octreotide (SANDOSTATIN): antidiarrheal, growth inhibitor, Rx: carcinoid tumor, acromegaly, intestinal tumors, diarrhea
OCUFLOX (ofloxacin): opthalmic anti-infective, Rx: conjunctivitis, corneal ulcers
Ofloxacin (FLOXIN): an antibiotic
Olanzapine (ZYPREXA): antipsychotic, Rx: psychosis
Olopatadine (PATANOL): antihistamine, Rx: allergic conjunctivitis
Olsalazine (DIPENTUM): salicylate, Rx: ulcerative colitis
Omeprazole (PRILOSEC): suppresses gastric acid secretion, Rx: ulcers, esophagitis, GERD
OMNARIS (ciclesonide): steroid anti-inflammatory nasal spray, Rx: allergies
OMNICEF (cefdinir): antibiotic, Rx: pneumonia, bronchitis
OMNIHIST LA (chlorpheniramine, phenylephrine, methscopalamine): antihistamine / decongestant
Ondansetron (ZOFRAN): antinauseant, Rx: N&V
Opium Alkaloids: narcotic analgesic / antidiarrheal
OPTICROM (cromolyn): antihistamine, mast cell stabilizer, Rx: conjunctivitis, keratitis
OPTIVAR (azelastine): antihistamine, anti-inflammatory, Rx: allergic conjunctivitis
ORAMORPH SR (morphine sulfate): narcotic analgesic
ORAP (pimozide): antipsychotic, Rx: motor & phonic tics
ORENCIA (abatacept): immune system inhibitor, Rx: rheumatoid arthritis
ORINASE (tolbutamide): oral hypoglycemic, Rx: diabetes
Orlistat (ZENICAL): lipase inhibitor, Rx: obesity
Orphenadrine (NORFLEX): analgesic, anticholinergic, Rx: pain relief
ORPHENGESIC (orphenadrine, aspirin, caffeine): analgesic, Rx: pain relief
ORTHO EVRA (norelgestromin, ethinyl estradiol): contraceptive

ORTHO TRI-CYCLEN-21, 28: an oral contraceptive
ORTHO-CEPT 21, 28: an oral contraceptive
ORTHO-CYCLEN-21, 28: an oral contraceptive
ORTHO-EST (estropipate): estrogen, Rx: menopause, osteoporosis
ORTHO-NOVUM: an oral contraceptive
OS-CAL: Calcium and Vitamin D supplement
OVCON an oral contraceptive
OVIDE (malathion): organophosphate insecticide, Rx: head lice
OVRAL: an oral contraceptive
OVRETTE (norgestrel): oral contraceptive
Oxandrolone (OXANDRIN): anabolic steroid, Rx: osteoporosis, promotes weight gain
Oxaprozin (DAYPRO): NSAID, Rx: arthritis
Oxazepam (SERAX): a benzodiazepine hypnotic
Oxcarbazepine (TRILEPTAL): anticonvulsant, Rx: partial seizures
Oxiconazole (OXISTAT): antifungal, Rx: skin infections
OXISTAT (oxiconazole): topical antifungal agent
OXSORALEN (methoxsalen): photosensitizer, Rx: repigmenting agent
Oxybutynin (DITROPAN): anticholinergic, antispasmodic, Rx: urinary incontinence
Oxycodone (PERCODAN): a narcotic analgesic
Oxycodone / ASP: narcotic analgesic + aspirin
Oxycodone w/ APAP (TYLOX): narcotic analgesic compound
OXYCONTIN (oxycodone): narcotic analgesic
OXYFAST (oxycodone): narcotic analgesic, Rx: pain relief
OXYIR (oxycodone): narcotic analgesic
Oxymetholone (ANADROL-50): anabolic steroid / androgen, Rx: anemia
Oxymorphone (NUMORPHAN): narcotic analgesic
Oxytetracycline (TERRAMYCIN): antibiotic, Rx: infections
OXYTROL (oxybutynin): urinary tract antispasmodic, Rx: incontinence

P

PACERONE (amiodarone): antiarrhythmic, Rx: cardiac arrhythmias
Paclitaxel (TAXOL): anticancer agent, Rx: ovarian cancer

Palivizumab (SYNAGIS): antiviral antibody, Rx: respiratory syncytial virus
PALLADONE (hydromorphone): narcotic analgesic
Pamabrom (VITELLE LURLINE PMS): diuretic, Rx: premenstrual syndrome
PAMELOR (nortriptyline): a tricyclic antidepressant
Pancrelipase (CREON 5): digestive enzyme replacement, Rx: pancreatitis, cystic fibrosis
PANHEMATIN (hemin): porphyrin inhibitor, Rx: porphyria related to menstrual cycle
Pantoprazole (PROTONIX): suppresses gastic acid, Rx: ulcers
PARAPLATIN (carboplatin): anti-cancer agent, Rx: ovarian CA
Paricalcitrol (ZEMPLAR): vitamin-D, Rx: hyperparathyroidism
PARNATE (tranylcypromine): MAO inhibitor, Rx: depression
Paroxetine (PAXIL): SSRI antidepressant, Rx: depression, OCD, anxiety, PTSD
PASER (aminosalicylic acid): bacteriostatic, Rx: TB
PATANOL (olopatadine): Rx: allergic conjunctivitis
PAXIL (paroxetine): antidepressant
PCE (erythromycin): an antibiotic
PEDIAFLOR (fluoride): mineral, Rx: osteoporosis, dental caries
PEDIAPRED (prednisolone): steroid, Rx: allergies, arthritis, MS
PEDIAZOLE: an antibiotic compound
PEDI-DRI (nystatin): antifungal antibiotic, Rx: fungal infection
PEGANONE (ethotoin): antiepileptic, rx: seizures
Pegaspargase (ONCASPAR): oncolytic agent, Rx: leukemia
PEGASYS (peginterferon alfa-2a): antiviral, Rx: Hepatitis C
Pemirolast (ALAMAST): antiinflammatory, Rx: allergic conjunctivitis
Pemoline (CYLERT): stimulant, Rx: ADHD, narcolepsy
Penbutolol (LEVATOL): beta blocker, Rx: HTN, angina
Penciclovir (DENAVIR): antiviral, Rx: herpes, cold sores
Penicillamine (CUPRIMINE): chelator, antirheumatic, Rx: heavy metal poisoning, Wilson's disease, arthritis, cystinuria
Penicillin: an antibiotic
PENTASA (mesalamine): for ulcerative colitis
Pentazocine (TALWIN): narcotic analgesic
Pentazocine & Naloxone (TALWIN NX): narcotic analgesic
Pentazocine/APAP: narcotic analgesic compound
Pentobarbital (NEMBUTAL): sedative / hypnotic, Rx: insomnia
Pentosan (ELMIRON): urinary tract analgesic, Rx: bladder pain
Pentostatin (NIPENT): chemotherapeutic, antibiotic, Rx: leukemia

Pentoxifylline (TRENTAL): reduces blood viscosity, improves circulation in peripheral vascular disease

PEPCID, PEPCID AC (famotidine): Histamine-2 blocker which inhibits gastric acid production, Rx: ulcers

PERCOCET (oxycodone, APAP): narcotic analgesic

PERCODAN (oxycodone, aspirin): narcotic analgesic

PERDIEM (psyllium): a bulk-forming laxative

Pergolide (PERMAX): dopamine receptor stimulator, Rx: Parkinson's disease

PERIACTIN (cyproheptadine): an antihistamine

PERI-COLACE (casanthranol, docusate): laxative / stool softener

Perindopril (ACEON): ACE inhibitor, Rx: HTN

PERIOSTAT (doxycycline): an antibiotic

PERMAX (pergolide): dopamine receptor stimulator, Rx: Parkinson's disease

Permethrin Lotion (ELIMITE): parasiticide, Rx: head lice

Perphenazine (TRILAFON): phenothiazine major tranquilizer

PERSANTINE (dipyridamole): cerebral & coronary vasodilator, Rx: CVA, angina

PFIZERPEN (penicillin): an antibiotic

Phenazopyridine (PYRIDIUM): urinary tract analgesic

Phenelzine (NARDIL): MAO inhibitor, Rx: depression, bulimia

PHENERGAN TABLETS (promethazine): sedative/antiemetic, Rx: rhinitis, urticaria, N&V

Pheniramine (NAPHCON-A): antihistamine, Rx: itching eyes

Phenobarbital: barbiturate sedative / anticonvulsant

PHENOL (carbolic acid): sore throat spray, Rx: sore throats

Phenoxybenzamine (DIBENZYLINE): alpha blocker, Rx: HTN, sweating

Phentermine (ADIPEX-P): amphetamine, Rx: obesity

Phenyl Salicylate (PROSED/DS): analgesic, Rx: urinary tract discomfort, cystitis, urethritis

Phenylephrine (NEO-SYNEPHRINE): decongestant, Rx: colds

PHENYTEK (phenytoin): anticonvulsant, Rx: seizures

Phenytoin (DILANTIN): anticonvulsant, Rx: epilepsy

PhosLo (calcium): phosphate reducer, Rx: renal failure

PHRENILIN, PHRENILIN FORTE (butalbital, acetaminophen): barbiturate sedative, analgesic, Rx: pain relief

Phytonadione (AQUAMEPHYTON): Vitamin K1, Rx: coagulation disorders

Pilocarpine (SALAGEN): cholinergic, Rx: dry mouth, Sjogren's syndrome

PIMA (potassium iodide): expectorant, Rx: asthma, bronchitis

Pimozide (ORAP): antipsychotic, Rx: Tourette's syndrome

Pindolol (VISKEN): beta blocker, Rx: HTN, angina
Pioglitazone (ACTOS): oral hypoglycemic, Rx: diabetes
Piperacillin (PIPRACIL): antibiotic
Pirbuterol (MAXAIR): beta bronchodilator, Rx: asthma, COPD
Piroxicam (FELDENE): NSAID analgesic, Rx: arthritis
PLAN B TABLETS (levonorgestrel): oral contraceptive, Rx: pregnancy prophylaxis
PLAQUENIL (hydroxychloroquine): an antimalarial agent
PLAVIX (clopidogrel): platelet inhibitor, Rx: MI, stroke, atherosclerosis
PLEGRIS-M (TM-BSPK): rectal ointment, Rx: anal itching
PLENDIL (felodipine): calcium blocker, Rx: HTN, angina
PLETAL (cilostazol): vasodilator, platelet inhibitor, Rx: leg cramps
PNEUMOTUSSIN (guaifenesin, hydrocodone): expectorant, narcotic antitussive, Rx: colds
PODOCON-25 (podophyllin): cytotoxic, Rx: venereal warts
Podofilox (CONDYLOX): destroys warts, Rx: anogenital warts
Podophyllin (PODOCON-25): cytotoxic agent, Rx: genital warts
Polymyxin (NEOSPORIN): an antibiotic
Polythiazide (RENESE): antihypertensive / diuretic, Rx: CHF, HTN
POLYTRIM (trimethoprim, polymyxin): antibacterial, Rx: eye infections
PONSTEL (mefenamic acid): NSAID analgesic
PORTIA (levonorgestrel, ethinyl estradiol): oral contraceptive
POTABA (aminobenzoate): antifibrotic, Rx: scleroderma, Peyronie's disease
Potassium Bicarbonate (KLOR-CON/EF): potassium supplement, Rx: dietary supplement
Potassium Chloride (K-TAB): potassium supplement
Potassium Citrate (UROCIT-K): increases urinary pH, increases citrate, Rx: kidney stones
Pramipexole (MIRAPEX): dopamine agonist, Rx: Parkinson's disease
PRAMOSONE (hydrocortisone, pramoxine): steroid antiinflammatory / anesthetic, Rx: dermatoses
Pramoxine (ANALPRAM HC): topical anesthetic, Rx: relief of itching, pain
PRANDIN (repaglinide): oral hypoglycemia, Rx: diabetes, hyperglycemia
PRAVACHOL (pravastatin): cholesterol reducer
Pravastatin (PRAVACHOL): statin, cholesterol reducer

PRAVIGARD PAC (pravastatin, ASA): statin cholesterol reducer, antiplatelet

PRAX (pramoxine): topical anesthetic, Rx: relief of itching, pain

Praziquantel (BILTRICIDE): antiparasitic, Rx: schistosome infections, liver flukes

Prazosin (MINIPRESS): alpha-1 blocker, vasodilator, Rx: HTN

PRECOSE (acarbose): delays carbohydrate digestion, Rx: diabetes mellitus

Prednisolone (ORAPRED): a steroid anti-inflammatory agent

Prednisone (DELTASONE): steroid anti-inflammatory agent

PREFEST (estradiol, norgestimate): hormones, Rx: menopause

PRELONE SYRUP (prednisolone): steroid anti-inflammatory

PRELU-2 (phendimetrazine): amphetamine appetite suppressant, Rx: obesity

PREMARIN: estrogens, Rx: menopause

PREMPHASE (estrogens, medroxyprogesterone): hormones, Rx: menopause, osteoporosis

PREMPRO (estrogens): hormone, Rx: menopause

PRENATE (vitamins): prenatal vitamins, Rx: nutritional supplement

PREVACID (lansoprazole): gastric acid pump inhibitor, Rx: ulcers, esophagitis

PREVALITE (cholestyramine): cholesterol reducer

PREVPAC (lansoprazole, amoxicillin, clarithromycin): inhibits gastric secretion, antibiotic, Rx: duodenal ulcers

PRIFTIN (rifapentine): antibiotic, Rx: tuberculosis

PRILOSEC (omeprazole): gastric acid pump inhibitor, Rx: ulcers, esophagitis

PRIMATENE MIST (epinephrine): bronchodilator, Rx: asthma

PRIMATENE Tablets (theophylline, ephedrine, phenobarbital) xanthine bronchodilator, Rx: asthma

PRIMAXIN (imipenem, cilastatin): antibiotic, Rx: infections

Primidone (MYSOLINE): anticonvulsant, Rx: epilepsy

PRINIVIL (lisinopril): ACE inhibitor, Rx: HTN, CHF

PRINZIDE (lisinopril, HCTZ): antihypertensive compound

PROAMATINE (midodrine): vasopressor, Rx: orthostatic hypotension

Probenecid (BENEMID): increases uric acid secretion in gout

Procainamide (PROCANBID): antiarrhythmic, Rx: PVCs

PROCANBID (procainamide): antiarrhythmic, Rx: PVCs

Procarbazine (MATULANE): antineoplastic, Rx: Hodgkin's disease

PROCARDIA, PROCARDIA XL (nifedipine): calcium channel blocker, Rx: angina, hypertension

Prochlorperazine (COMPAZINE): phenothiazine antiemetic
PROCRIT (epoetin alfa): stimulates red blood cell production, Rx: anemia, renal failure, HIV
PROCTOCORT (hydrocortisone): steroid anti-inflammatory, Rx: inflammation, itching
PROCTOCREAM-HC (hydrocortisone): steroid anti-inflammatory, Rx: inflammation, itching
PROCTOFOAM-HC (hydrocortisone): steroid anti-inflammatory, Rx: inflammation, itching
Progesterone (CRINONE): fertility hormone
PROGRAF (tacrolimus): immunosuppressant, Rx: liver and kidney transplants
PROLASTIN (alpha-1 proteinase inhibitor): Rx: alpha-1 antitrypsin deficiency, emphysema
Promethazine (PHENERGAN): sedative / antiemetic
PROMETRIUM (progesterone): fertility hormone, Rx: infertile women, amenorrhea, endometrial hyperplasia
Propafenone (RYTHMOL): beta blocker, antiarrhythmic, Rx: PSVT, paroxysmal atrial fibrillation
Propantheline: anticholinergic, inhibits gastric acid secretion, Rx: peptic ulcers
PROPECIA (finasteride): dihydrotestosterone inhibitor, Rx: hair loss, baldness
Propoxyphene (DARVON): narcotic analgesic
Propranolol (INDERAL): beta blocker, Rx: HTN, prophylaxis of: angina, cardiac dysrhythmias, AMI, and migraine H/A
PROSCAR (finasteride): Rx: prostatic hypertrophy
PROSED/DS (methenamine, phenyl salicylate, methylene blue, benzoic acid, atropine, hyoscyamine): bactericidal, analgesic, antiseptic, Rx: urinary tract infections
PROSOM (estazolam): hypnotic, Rx: insomnia
Protease (ARCO-LASE): digestive enzyme, Rx: poor digestion
PROTONIX (pantoprazole): proton pump inhibitor, Rx: ulcers
Protriptyline (VIVACTIL): tricyclic antidepressant, Rx: depression
PROVENTIL (albuterol): beta-2 bronchodilator, Rx: COPD, asthma
PROVENTIL HFA (albuterol): beta-2 bronchodilator, Rx: asthma
PROVERA (medroxyprogesterone): hormone, Rx: amenorrhea
PROVIGIL (modafinil): wakefulness-promoting agent, Rx: narcolepsy, daytime sleepiness
PROZAC (fluoxetine): a heterocyclic antidepressant
Pseudoephedrine (HALOTUSSIN): decongestant, Rx: colds

PSORCON E (diflorasone): steroid anti-inflammatory, Rx: dermatoses
Psyllium (METAMUCIL): fiber laxative, Rx: constipation
PULMICORT Turbuhaler (budesonide): steroid antiinflammatory, Rx: asthma
PULMOZYME (dornase alfa or DNase): lytic enzyme which dissolves infected lung secretions, Rx: cystic fibrosis
PURINETHOL (mercaptopurine): antileukemia agent
Pyrazinamide (RIFATER): antibacterial, Rx: TB
PYRIDIUM (phenazopyridine): urinary tract analgesic
Pyridostigmine (MESTINON): anticholinesterase, Rx: myasthenia gravis
Pyridoxine (vitamin B-6): vitamin, Rx: dietary supplement, INH poisoning, sideroblastic anemia, seizures in neonates
Pyrilamine (ATROHIST): antihistamine, Rx: colds, allergies
Pyrimethamine (DARAPRIM): antiparasitic, Rx: toxoplasmosis, malaria

Q

Quetiapine (SEROQUEL): antipsychotic, Rx: psychosis
Quinapril (ACCUPRIL): ACE inhibitor, Rx: HTN, CHF
Quinapril -HCTZ (Quinaretic): ACE inhibitor, diuretic, Rx: HTN
QUINARETIC (quinapril -HCTZ): ACE inhibitor, diuretic, Rx: HTN
QUINIDEX (quinidine): antiarrhythmic, Rx: supraventricular and ventricular dysrhythmias
Quinidine gluconate, sulfate (quinidine): antiarrhythmic, Rx: supraventricular and ventricular dysrhythmias
Quinine: antimalarial, Rx: malaria
Quinupristin/Dalfopristin (SYNERCID): antimicrobials
QUIXIN (levofloxacin): ocular anti-infective, Rx: conjunctivitis
QVAR (beclomethasone): steroid anti-inflammatory, Rx: asthma

R

Raloxifene (EVISTA): Rx: osteoporosis prevention
Ramipril (ALTACE): ACE inhibitor, Rx: HTN
RANEXA (ranolazine): antianginal, Rx: chronic angina
Ranitidine (ZANTAC): histamine-2 blocker, Rx: ulcers
RAPAMUNE (sirolimus): immunosuppressive, Rx: prevents organ transplant rejection
REBETROL (ribavirin): antiviral, Rx: Hepatitis C
REBETRON (interferon alfa, ribavirin): antivirals, Rx: Hepatitis C

Rebif (interferon-beta-1a): antiviral, Rx: multiple sclerosis
RECOMBINATE (Factor VIII): clotting agent, Rx: hemophilia
REGLAN (metoclopramide): improves gastric emptying,
Rx: heartburn, ulcers
RELAFEN (nabumetone): NSAID, Rx: arthritis
RELENZA (zanamivir) an antiviral, Rx: influenza
RELPAX (eletriptan): antimigraine, Rx: migraine headaches
REMERON (mirtazapine): antidepressant, Rx: depression
REMICADE (infliximab): neutralizes tumor necrosis factor,
Rx: Crohn's disease
REMINYL (galantamine): acetylcholinesterase inhibitor,
Rx: Alzheimer's disease
RENACIDIN (citric acid, glucono-delta-lactone, magnesium
carbonate): antiurolithic, Rx: dissolves urinary tract stones
RENAGEL (sevelamer): phosphate binder, Rx: renal disease,
osteoporosis
RENESE (polythiazide): antihypertensive/diuretic, Rx: CHF,
HTN
RENOVA (tretinoin): an anti-acne, anti-wrinkle agent
Repaglinide (PRANDIN): stimulates insulin release,
Rx: diabetes
REPRONEX (mentropins): fertility drug, induces ovulation
REQUIP (ropinirole): dopaminergic, Rx: Parkinson's disease,
restless legs syndrome
RESCRIPTOR (delavirdine): antiviral, Rx: HIV
RESTASIS (cyclosporine eye drops): immunosuppressive,
increases tear volume
RESTORIL (temazepam): a benzodiazepine hypnotic
RESTYLANE (hyaluronan): anti-inflammmatory / wrinkle
remover, Rx: facial wrinkles
RETIN-A (tretinoin): an anti-acne, anti-wrinkle agent
RETROVIR (zidovudine): antiviral agent, Rx: HIV(AIDS) virus
REVATIO (sildenafil): vasodilator, Rx: pulmonary artery
hypertension
REYATAZ (atazanavir): protease inhibitor, antiviral, Rx: HIV /
AIDS
RHINOCORT (budesonide): corticosteroid, Rx: allergic rhinitis
Ribavirin (REBETROL): antiviral, Rx: viral infections
RIFADIN (rifampin): antibiotic, Rx: tuberculosis, meningitis
RIFAMATE (rifampin, isoniazid): antibiotics, Rx: tuberculosis
Rifampin (RIFADIN): antibiotic, Rx: tuberculosis, meningitis
Rifapentine (PRIFTIN): antibiotic, Rx: tuberculosis
RIFATER (isoniazid, rifampin, pyrazinamide): antibiotic, Rx: TB
RILUTEK (riluzole): Rx: amyotrophic lateral sclerosis(ALS)
RIMACTANE (rifampin): antibiotic, Rx: TB, meningitis

Risedronate (ACTONEL): bone stabilizer, Rx: Paget's disease
RISPERDAL (risperidone): antipsychotic, Rx: schizophrenia, autism
Risperidone (RISPERDAL): antipsychotic, Rx: schizophrenia
RITALIN, RITALIN-LA (methylphenidate): a stimulant, Rx: attention deficit hyperactivity disorder in children, narcolepsy
Ritonavir (NORVIR): antiviral, Rx: HIV / AIDS
Rivastigmine (EXELON): cholinesterase inhibitor, Rx: Alzheimer's disease
RMS (morphine sulfate): narcotic analgesic suppositories
ROBAXIN (methocarbamol): sedative, Rx: painful musculoskeletal conditions
ROBINUL, ROBINUL FORTE (glycopyrrolate): anticholinergic, Rx: peptic ulcers
ROBITUSSIN (guaifenesin): expectorant
ROCALTROL (calcitrol): vitamin D analog, Rx: hypocalcemia, bone disease
ROCEPHIN (ceftriaxone): an antibiotic
ROFERON-A (interferon): immunoadjuvant, Rx: hairy cell leukemia, AIDS-related Kaposi's sarcoma
ROGAINE (minoxidil): topical hair growing agent, Rx: baldness
Ropinirole (REQUIP): dopaminergic, Rx: Parkinson's disease
Rosiglitazone (AVANDIA): oral hypoglycemic, Rx: diabetes
ROWASA (mesalamine): anti-inflammatory, Rx: colitis, proctitis
ROXANOL 100 (morphine): narcotic analgesic
ROXICET (oxycodone, APAP): narcotic analgesic compound
ROXICODONE (oxycodone): narcotic analgesic
ROZEREM (ramelteon): hypnotic, Rx: insomnia
ROZEX (metronidazole): antibacterial, antiprotozoal, Rx: rosacea
RUM-K (potassium): potassium supplement
RYNATAN (phenylephrine, chlorpheniramine, pyrilamine): antihistamine / decongestant compound
RYNATUSS: antitussive / decongestant / antihistamine
RYTHMOL, RYTHMOL SR (propafenone): antiarrhythmic, Rx: severe ventricular dysrhythmias such as ventricular tachycardia, atrial fibrillation

S

SAIZEN (somatropin): growth hormone
SALAGEN (pilocarpine): parasympathomimetic, Rx: glaucoma
Salicylic acid (SAL-ACID), Rx: removes warts

Salmeterol (SEREVENT): ß-2 bronchodilator, Rx: asthma, COPD
SALPLANT Gel (salicylic acid): for removal of common warts
SANDIMMUNE (cyclosporine): immunosuppressant agent, Rx: prophylaxis of rejection of transplanted organs
SANDOSTATIN (octreotide): antidiarrheal, growth inhibitor, Rx: carcinoid tumor, acromegaly, intestinal tumors, diarrhea
Saquinavir (FORTOVASE): antiviral, Rx: HIV / AIDS
SARAFEM (fluoxetine): antidepressant, Rx: PMDD [premenstrual dysphoric disorder], depression, panic disorder, bulemia
SARAPIN (Pitcher Plant extract): analgesic, Rx: nerve block for sciatic pain, neuritis, neuralgia
Scopolamine (DONNATAL): antispasmodic / sedative
SEASONALE (levonorgestrel, estradiol): extended-cycle oral contraceptive
SEDAPAP (butalbital, APAP): sedative/analgesic, Rx: tension H/A
Selegiline (ELDEPRYL): MAO inhibitor, Rx: Parkinson's disease
Selenium (SELSUN BLUE): mineral, Rx: seborrhea, dandruff
SEMPREX-D (acrivastine, pseudoephedrine): antihistamine / decongestant
Senna Extract (SENOKOT): laxative, Rx: constipation
SENOKOT (senna fruit extract): a laxative
SENOKOT XTRA (senna extract): laxative, Rx: constipation
SENOKOT-S (senna, docusate): laxative / stool softener, Rx: constipation
SEPTRA, SEPTRA DS (trimethoprim, sulfamethoxazole): antibacterial compound, Rx: UTI, ear infection, bronchitis
SERENTIL (mesoridazine): a major tranquilizer
SEREVENT (salmeterol): ß-2 bronchodilator, Rx: asthma, COPD
Sermorelin (GEREF): growth hormone
SEROPHENE (clomiphene): induces ovulation
SEROQUEL (quetiapine): antipsychotic, Rx: schizophrenia, depression
SEROSTIM (somatropin): hormone, Rx: AIDS wasting
SERPACWA (perfluoroalkylpolyether, polytetrafluoroethylene): Skin Exposure Reduction Paste Against Chemical Warfare Agents: Rx: chemical warfare
Sertraline (ZOLOFT): antidepressant, Rx: depression, panic disorder, obsessive-compulsive disorder
SERZONE (nefazodone): antidepressant, Rx: depression

SILVADENE (silver sulfadiazine): topical antimicrobial agent, Rx: infection prophylaxis for burns of the skin

SIMPLY COUGH LIQUID (dextromethorphan): antitussive

Simvastatin (Zocor): cholesterol reducer

SINEMET CR (carbidopa, levodopa): dopamine precursors, Rx: Parkinson's Disease

SINEQUAN (doxepin): a tricyclic antidepressant

SINGULAIR (montelukast): Rx: asthma

SINUVENT (phenylpropanolamine, guaifenesin): decongestant / expectorant

SKELAXIN (metaxalone): sedative / analgesic

SLO-NIACIN (niacin): reduces serum cholesterol

SOMA (carisoprodol): sedative / antispasmodic

SOMA Compound (carisoprodol, aspirin): sedative / antispasmodic / analgesic, Rx: muscle spasm

Somatropin (NORDITROPIN): growth hormone, Rx: growth failure

SONATA (zaleplon): hypnotic, Rx: insomnia

SORIATANE (acitretin): retinoid, Rx: psoriasis

Sotalol (BETAPACE): ß-blocker, Rx: HTN, angina, arrhythmias

SPECTAZOLE (econazole): antifungal agent

SPECTRACEF (cefditoren): an antibiotic

SPIRIVA (tiotropium): anticholinergic bronchodilator, Rx: COPD

Spironolactone (ALDACTONE): potassium-sparing diuretic

Spironolactone & HCTZ: diuretics, Rx: HTN

SPORANOX (itraconazole): an antifungal

SPRINTEC (norgestimate, estradiol): oral contraceptive

SSKI (potassium iodide): an expectorant

STADOL NS (butorphanol): a narcotic analgesic

STAGESIC (hydrocodone, APAP): narcotic analgesic compound

STALEVO (levodopa/carbidopa/entacapone): dopamine precursors, Rx: Parkinson's disease

STATUSS DM (dextromethorphan, phenylephrine, chlorpheniramine): non-narcotic antitussive, decongestant, antihistamine compound

STATUSS GREEN (hydrocodone, phenylephrine, pseudoephedrine, pyrilamine, chlorpheniramine): narcotic antitussive, decongestant, antihistamine compund

Stavudine d4T (ZERIT): antiviral, Rx: HIV

STELAZINE (trifluoperazine): a major tranquilizer

STRATTERA (atomoxetine): stimulant, Rx: ADHD

Streptomycin: an antibiotic

STRIANT (testosterone): androgen, Rx: adult male hypogonadism

168

STROMECTOL (ivermectin): anti-parasite, Rx: intestinal nematodes
SUBOXONE (buprenorphine, naloxone): narcotic analgesic, narcotic antagonist, Rx: opiate addiction
SUBUTEX (buprenorphine): narcotic analgesic, Rx: opiate addiction
Sucralfate (CARAFATE): anti-ulcer agent, Rx: duodenal ulcers
Sufentanil: narcotic analgesic / anesthetic
SULAR (nisoldipine): calcium channel blocker, Rx: HTN
Sulfamethoxazole (SEPTRA): a bacteriostatic, Rx: UTI
Sulfanilamide (AVC): anti-infective, Rx: candida
Sulfisoxazole (PEDIAZOLE): a bacteriostatic agent, Rx: UTI
Sulindac (CLINORIL): NSAID analgesic, Rx: arthritis
Sumatriptan (IMITREX): Rx: migraine H/A
SUPRAX (cefixime): broad spectrum antibiotic
SURMONTIL (trimipramine): a tricyclic antidepressant
SUSTIVA (efavirenz): antiviral, Rx: HIV, AIDS
SYMBYAX (olanzapine and fluoxetine) psychotropic, antidepressant, Rx: bipolar disorder
SYMMETREL (amantadine): an antiparkinsonian / antiviral
SYNAGIS (palivizumab): antiviral antibody, Rx: respiratory syncytial virus
SYNALGOS-DC (dihydrocodeine, aspirin, caffeine): narcotic analgesic compound
SYNAREL (naferelin): gonadotropin-releasing hormone, Rx: endometriosis, precocious puberty, decreased gonadal steroids, dysmenorrhea
SYNTHROID (levothyroxine): thyroid hormone
SYPRINE (trientine): copper chelator, Rx: Wilson's disease

T

TABLOID (thioguanine): purine analog, Rx: leukemia
TAGAMET (cimetidine): inhibits gastric acid secretion, Rx: ulcers
TALACEN (pentazocine, APAP): narcotic analgesic
TALWIN NX (pentazocine, naloxone): narcotic analgesic
TAMBOCOR (flecainide): ventricular antiarrhythmic
TAMIFLU (oseltamivir) an antiviral, Rx: influenza
Tamoxifen (NOLVADEX): anticancer agent, Rx: breast CA
TAO (troleandomycin): antibiotic, Rx: pneumonia, URI
TAPAZOLE (methimazole): antithyroid, Rx: hyperthyroidism
TARKA (trandolapril, verapamil): ACE inhibitor / calcium blocker, Rx: HTN
TASMAR (tolcapone): COMT inhibitor, Rx: Parkinson's disease

TEGRETOL, TEGRETOL XR (carbamazepine): anticonvulsant
Telmisartan (MICARDIS): ACE inhibitor, Rx: HTN
Temazepam (RESTORIL): benzodiazepine hypnotic
TEMOVATE (clobetasol): steroid anti-inflammatory
TENORMIN (atenolol): ß-1 blocker, Rx: dysrhythmias, HTN, angina, MI prophylaxis
TENUATE (diethylpropion): stimulant, appetite suppressant, Rx: obesity
Terazosin (HYTRIN): alpha-1 blocker antihypertensive
Terbinafine (LAMISIL): antifungal, Rx: nail fungus, ringworm
Terbutaline (BRETHINE): bronchodilator, Rx: asthma, COPD
Terconazole (TERAZOL): antimicrobial
TERRA-CORTRIL (hydrocortisone, oxytetracycline): steroid anti-inflammatory, antibiotic, Rx: ocular infections
TESSALON (benzonatate): a non-narcotic cough suppressant
Testosterone (ANDRODERM): androgenizing hormone
TESTRED (methyltestosterone): androgenizing hormone
Tetracycline (HELIDAC): an antibiotic
TEVETEN (eprosartan): angiotensin II inhibitor, Rx: HTN
TEVETEN HCT (eprosartan, HCT): angiotensin II inhibitor, diuretic, Rx: HTN
Thalidomide (THALOMID): immunosuppressant, Rx: HIV, leprosy
THALOMID (thalidomide): immunosuppressant, Rx: HIV, leprosy
THEO-24 (theophylline): bronchodilator, Rx: asthma, COPD
THEOLAIR (theophylline): bronchodilator, Rx: asthma, COPD
Theophylline (UNIPHYL): bronchodilator, Rx: asthma, COPD
THERA-GESIC (salicylate): topical NSAID analgesic, Rx: arthritis
Thiabendazole (MINTEZOL): antiparasitic, Rx: pinworm, roundworm, trichinosis
Thiamine (vitamin B-1): vitamin supplement
Thioguanine (TABLOID): anticancer agent, Rx: leukemia
THIOLA (tiopronin): cysteine-depleting agent, Rx: kidney stone prevention
Thioridazine: major tranquilizer
Thiothixene (NAVANE): major tranquilizer
THORAZINE (chlorpromazine): a major tranquilizer
THYROLAR (liotrix): thyroid hormone
Tiagabine (GABITRIL): antiepileptic, Rx: partial seizures
TIAZAC (diltiazem): calcium blocker, Rx: HTN, angina, PSVT
Ticarcillin (TIMENTIN): antibiotic, Rx: infection
TICLID (ticlopidine): platelet inhibitor, Rx: stroke prophylaxis
TIGAN (trimethobenzamide): an antiemetic

TIKOSYN (dofetilide): antiarrhythmic, Rx: atrial fibrillation
TILADE (nedocromil): anti-inflammatory, Rx: asthma
TIMENTIN (ticarcillin / clavulanate): antibiotic compound
TIMOLIDE (timolol, HCTZ): ß-blocker / antihypertensive / diuretic
Timolol (BLOCADREN) ß-blocker, Rx: HTN, angina, arrhythmias
TIMOPTIC (timolol): ß-blocker, Rx: glaucoma
Tizanidine (ZANAFLEX): alpha blocker, Rx: spasticity
TOBI Solution for Inhalation (tobramycin): antibiotic, Rx: cystic fibrosis
TOBRADEX (tobramycin, dexamethasone): antibiotic / steroid, Rx: eye infection / inflammation
TOFRANIL, TOFRANIL PM (imipramine): a tricyclic antidepressant
Tolazamide: oral hypoglycemic, Rx: diabetes
Tolbutamide: oral hypoglycemic, Rx: diabetes
Tolmetin: NSAID analgesic
Tolterodine (DETROL): urinary bladder antispasmodic, Rx: overactive bladder
TOPAMAX (topiramate): anticonvulsant, Rx: seizures
TOPROL-XL (metoprolol): cardioselective beta blocker, Rx: HTN, angina, arrhythmias
TORADOL (ketorolac): NSAID analgesic
TRACLEER (bosentan): endothelin receptor antagonist, Rx: pulmonary hypertension
Tramadol (ULTRAM): analgesic
TRANDATE (labetalol): beta blocker, Rx: hypertension
Trandolapril (MAVIK): ACE inhibitor, Rx: HTN, CHF
TRANSDERM-SCOP (scopolamine): anticholinergic antiemetic, Rx: motion sickness prophylaxis
TRANXENE T-TAB, TRANXENE SD (clorazepate): benzodiazepine hypnotic, Rx: anxiety, seizures
TRAUMEEL: anti-inflammatory, Rx: arthritis
TRASYLOL (aprotinin): reduces intraocular pressure, Rx: glaucoma
Trazodone (DESYREL): an antidepressant
TRECATOR-SC (ethionamide): bacteriostatic, Rx: tuberculosis
TRENTAL (pentoxifylline): reduces blood viscosity, improves circulation in peripheral vascular disease
Tretinoin (RETIN-A): an anti-acne, anti-wrinkle agent
TRIAM/HCTZ (triamcinolone, hydrochlorothiazide): steroid antiinflammatory, diuretic
Triamcinolone (AZMACORT): steroid anti-inflammatory
Triamterene w/ HCTZ (DYAZIDE): antihypertensive / diuretic

Triazolam (HALCION): benzodiazepine hypnotic, Rx: insomnia

TRICOR (fenofibrate): lipid regulator, Rx: hyperlipidemia

TRIEMOL (ameplidnarmag): antiarrhythmic, Rx: cardiac arrhythmias

Trifluoperazine (STELAZINE): a major tranquilizer

TRIGLIDE (fenofibrate): lipid reducer, Rx: high cholesterol

Trihexyphenidyl (ARTANE): antispasmodic, Rx: Parkinson's Disease

TRILEPTAL (oxcarbazepine): anticonvulsant, Rx: partial seizures

TRI-LEVLEN: an oral contraceptive

TRILISATE (salicylate): anti-inflammatory / analgesic

Trimethoprim (SEPTRA): an antibiotic

Trimethoprim & Sulfamethoxazole: antibacterials, Rx: UTI, ear infection, bronchitis

TRI-NORINYL 28: an oral contraceptive

TRINSICON (vitamins): anti-anemia compound

TRIOVAN (trovafloxacin): an antibacterial

TRIPHASIL: an oral contraceptive

TRISENOX (arsenic): suppresses bone marrow, Rx: leukemia

TRIZIVIR (abacavir, lamivudine, zidovudine): antivirals, Rx: HIV infection

TRUSOPT (dorzolamide): Rx: glaucoma, reduction of IOP

TUSSAFED HC (hydrocodone, phenylephrine, guaifenesin): narcotic antitussive / decongestant / expectorant

TUSSIONEX (hydrocodone, chlorpheniramine): narcotic antitussive / antihistamine, Rx: coughs, allergies, the cold

TYLENOL w/ Codeine (APAP, codeine): narcotic analgesic

TYZEKA (telbivudine): antiviral, Rx: Hepatitis B

U

ULTRABROM, ULTRABROM PD (brompheniramine, pseudoephedrine): antihistamine / decongestant

ULTRACET (tramadol, APAP): narcotic analgesic compound

ULTRAM (tramadol): analgesic, Rx: pain relief

ULTRASE, ULTRASE MT (pancreatic enzymes): Rx: cystic fibrosis, pancreatitis

ULTRAVATE (halobetasol): steroid anti-inflammatory, Rx: pruritus

UNIPHYL (theophylline): bronchodilator, Rx: asthma, COPD

UNIRETIC (moexepril, HCTZ): ACE inhibitor / diuretic, Rx: HTN

UNISOM (doxylamine): antihistamine sedative, Rx: insomnia

UNITHROID (levothyroxine): thyroid hormone supplement

UNIVASC (moexipril): ACE inhibitor, Rx: HTN

URECHOLINE (bethanechol): increases bladder tone, Rx: urinary retention

URIMAX (methenamine, salicylate, methylene blue, hyoscyamine): urinary tract antiseptic, analgesic, antispasmodic, Rx: UTI

URISED (methenamine, methylene blue, salicylate, atropine, hyoscyamine): antiseptic / analgesic /antispasmodic, Rx: UTI

UROAXTRAL (alfuzosin): smooth muscle relaxer, Rx: prostatic hypertrophy

UROCIT-K (potassium citrate): urinary alkalinizer, Rx: kidney stones

URO-KP-NEUTRAL (dipotassium phosphate): urinary acidifier, antiurolithic, Rx: UTI, kidney stones

URO-MAG (magnesium): magnesium supplement

UROQID ACID No. 2 (methenamine): bactericide, Rx: UTI

Ursodiol (ACTIGALL): bile acid which dissolves gall stones

V

Valacyclovir (VALTREX): antiviral, Rx: herpes, shingles

VALCYTE (valganciclovir): antiviral, Rx: cytomegalovirus

VALIUM (diazepam): a benzodiazepine hypnotic

Valproic acid (DEPAKENE): anticonvulsant, Rx: seizures

Valrubicin (VALSTAR): anticancer agent, Rx: bladder cancer

Valsartan (DIOVAN): angiotensin II inhibitor, Rx: HTN

VALTREX (valaciclovir): antiviral, Rx: herpes, shingles

VANCENASE, VANCENASE AQ (beclomethasone): steroid anti-inflammatory agent, Rx: allergic rhinitis, nasal polyps

VANCOCIN (vancomycin): an antibiotic

Vancomycin (VANCOCIN): antibiotic, Rx: colitis

VANTIN (cefpodoxime): an antibiotic

VASERETIC (enalapril, HCTZ): antihypertensive / diuretic

VASOTEC (enalaprilat): an ACE inhibitor, Rx: HTN, CHF

VELOSULIN (insulin): hypoglycemic, Rx: diabetes mellitus

Venlafaxine (EFFEXOR): an antidepressant

VENTOLIN (albuterol): ß-2 bronchodilator, Rx: asthma, COPD

Verapamil (ISOPTIN): calcium blocker, Rx: angina, PSVT, HTN

VERELAN, VERELAN PM (verapamil): calcium blocker, Rx: angina, hypertension, PSVT prophylaxis, headache

VERMOX (mebendazole): anthelminthic, Rx: intestinal worms

VESANOID (tretinoin): anticancer agent, Rx: leukemia

VFEND (voriconazole): antifungal, Rx: fungal infections

VIAGRA (sildenafil): Rx: male erectile dysfunction

VIBRAMYCIN (doxycycline): an antibiotic

VIBRA-TABS (doxycycline): an antibiotic

VICODIN HP, VICODIN ES (hydrocodone, APAP): narcotic analgesic / antitussive compound
VICODIN TUSS (hydrocodone, guaifenesin): narcotic analgesic / antitussive expectorant compound
VICON FORTE: vitamins
VICOPROFEN (hydrocodone, ibuprofen): narcotic analgesic comp.
VIDEX (didanosine): an antiviral, Rx: AIDS
VIOKASE (pancreatic enzymes): Rx: cystic fibrosis, pancreatitis
VIRACEPT (nelfinavir): protease inhibitor antiviral, Rx: HIV
VIRAMUNE (nevirapine): antiviral, Rx: HIV
VIRAZOLE (ribavirin): an antiviral, Rx: chronic Hepatitis C
VIREAD (tenofovir): nucleoside analog antiviral, Rx: HIV /AIDS
VIRILON (methyltestosterone): androgen / masculinizing hormone
VISTARIL (hydroxyzine): antiemetic / antihistamine / sedative
VITAFOL OB: multivitamins and minerals
VITORIN (exetimibe, simvastatin): lowers cholesterol
VIVACTIL (protriptyline): tricyclic antidepressant
VIVELLE (estradiol), Rx: osteoporosis, menopausal symptoms
VOLMAX (albuterol): ß-2 bronchodilator, Rx: asthma, COPD
VOLTAREN, VOLTAREN XR (diclofenac): NSAID analgesic
VOSPIRE ER (albuterol): beta-2 bronchodilator, Rx: asthma, COPD

W

Warfarin (COUMADIN): anticoagulant, Rx: A-Fib, MI, thrombosis
WELCHOL (colesevelam): lowers serum cholesterol
WELLBUTRIN, WELLBUTRIN SR (bupropion): an antidepressant

X

XANAX, XANAX XR (alprazolam): a benzodiazepine hypnotic
XELODA (capecitabine): oral anticancer agent, Rx: breast CA
XENICAL (orlistat): lipase inhibitor, Rx: obesity
XIFAXAN (rifaximin): antibiotic, Rx: traveller's diarrhea
XOPENEX (levalbuterol): ß-2 bronchodilator, Rx: asthma, COPD

Drugs

XYREM (sodium oxybate-GHB): CNS depressant,
Rx: cataplexy

Y

YASMIN 28 (drospirenone, estradiol): oral contraceptive
YAZ (drospirenone, estradiol): hormones, Rx: premenstrual
dysphoric disorder
YODOXIN (iodoquinol): amebicide, Rx: intestinal amebiasis
Yohimbine (APHRODYNE): alpha blocker, Rx: impotence

Z

ZADITOR (ketotifen): antihistamine, anti-inflammatory,
Rx: allergic conjunctivitis
Zalcitabine (HIVID): antiviral, Rx: HIV, AIDS
Zaleplon (SONATA): anxiolytic, hypnotic, Rx: insomnia
ZANAFLEX (tizanidine): muscle relaxant, Rx: muscle spasticity
ZARONTIN (ethosuximide): anticonvulsant, Rx: absence Sz
ZAROXOLYN (metolazone): antihypertensive / diuretic
ZEBETA (bisoprolol): ß-blocker antihypertensive
ZELNORM (tegaserod): stimulates peristalsis, Rx: constipation,
IBS
ZEMPLAR (paricalcitol): vitamin D analog,
Rx: hyperparathyroidism
ZERIT (stavudine d4T): antiviral, Rx: HIV
ZESTORETIC (lisinopril, HCTZ): ACE inhibitor / diuretic,
Rx: HTN
ZESTRIL (lisinopril): ACE inhibitor, Rx: HTN, CHF
ZETIA (ezetimibe): lipid lowering agent, Rx: high cholesterol
ZIAC (bisoprolol, HCTZ): antihypertensive / diuretic, Rx: HTN
ZIAGEN (abacavir): antiviral, Rx: HIV
ZIANA (clindamycin, tretinoin): antibiotic, retinoid, Rx: acne
Zidovudine (AZT - RETROVIR): an antiviral agent, Rx: HIV /
AIDS
ZINACEF (cefuroxime): antibiotic, Rx: infections
ZINECARD (dexrazoxane): cardioprotective agent, chelating
agent, Rx: cardiomyopathy
ZITHROMAX (azithromycin): an antibiotic
ZOCOR (simvastatin): cholesterol reducer
ZOFRAN (ondansetron): antinauseant, Rx: chemotherapy
ZOLADEX (goserelin) gonadotropin-releasing hormone
agonist, Rx: endometriosis
ZOLOFT (sertraline): antidepressant
Zolpidem (AMBIEM): hypnotic, Rx: insomnia
ZOMIG (zolmitriptan): Rx: migraine headache